JesseA's

My 'Mythical Tongue'

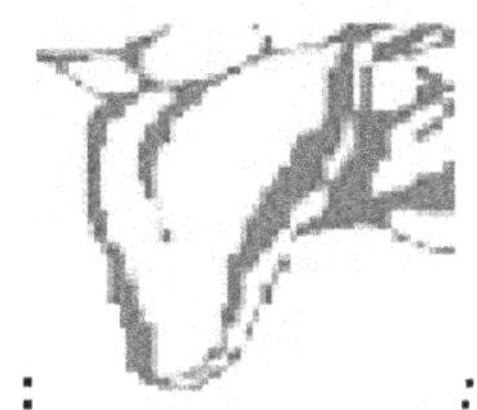

Jesse George Steven Alecho

Publisher

Alawi Books Ltd

Book - ISBN 978-0-9929462-9-6

Publisher:

Alawi Books ltd

Website at:
www.tboah.com

Contacts:
Email: ofano759@gmail.com

Tel: [+44] 07767157506

Ordering information:

My Mythical Tongue is available as a hard copy and e-copy from Amazon Books.

Cover design, Layout and Illustrations: Jesse G.S. Alecho

Thanks / Inspiration

Bearing the topic in mind, as you happen to read this book you will realise that I have had a bunch of inspirations and those to thank for my own existence. At the onset, I want to state clearly that the more prominent *'Mythical Tongue'* is a 'She'. The Tongue is in the mother. The intertwined umbilical cord creates the very co-existence of the mother tongue in the eyes of the mother's world. I would, therefore, like to thank my mother who laboured with me from cradle to this day. In her eyes, I have never stopped being her 'Child', I will never cease being someone's child.

Next, she once told me one thing when I asked her that I wanted to go to Kampala City. She told me that if you want 'good things' you have to get 'a pen and paper'. I did exactly that and flew the nest, by the time I winked, I was in the United Kingdom; and, since, have made a home here. However, I still left her deep in our village home of Lwala P'Obona, Uganda, where she told me to get a pen and paper, still toiling to make ends meet. Still scrubbing the soot infested pots with her dry scaly hands. Still tiling the land with her trodden hoe. That is the touch of a mother's well-being stated in a mother tongue inscribed as a 'She'.

At least, I must thank you Besimesi Nyafwono Ochwo Alecho; for being there for me in the thick and thin of the moment. The only thing I will not allow you to do is to read this book. I will not *'mythically'* break your heart because I signed a *'mythical non-disclosure mythical agreement'* and it is embedded in my *'mythical Sin'*.

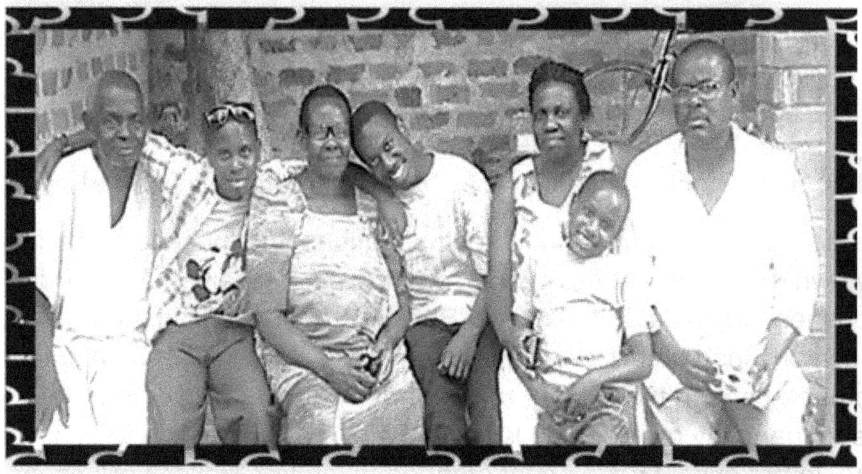

I give gratitude to my family from left to right. The Late Baba Ochiengh Alecho *[famously referred to as 'Councillor']* who gave me a shoulder to be carried on and was there for me from infancy after my dad passed away. He put me in line to be straight and narrow and never spared the rod. He was always upfront whenever he felt I was going astray and needed guidance. He directed me to the real world and not the imagery of the world.

To my late Son, Israel Ochwo Alecho, who from childhood, was my pillar sometimes in hours of need a tap on my shoulder was an assurance of his presence.

To my mother Besimesi Nyafwono Ochwo Alecho, whom I have already expressed my thanks.

To my Son Arnold Ochiengh Alecho whose presence in me has been a reassurance that I am in safe hands.

To my wife Agnes Athieno Alecho who has been there for me in whatever environments and episodes she has not faltered.

To Jerokam Stephen Alecho who will forever remind me of my late brother's existence in me. He plays around with me as if we are indeed Siblings. I am forever grateful as the *'My Mythical Tongue'* reverberates.

["Gratitude turns what we have into enough, and more. It turns denial into acceptance, chaos into order, confusion into clarity... it makes sense of our past, brings peace for today, and creates a vision for tomorrow. " Melody Beattie]

Contents

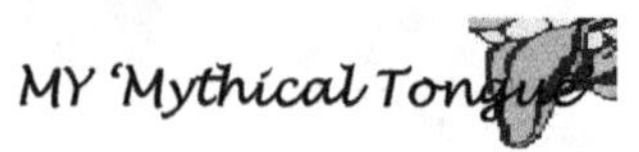

Glossary

- Baganda - describes the nationalities occupying Buganda, part of the wider Ntu person.
- Buganda - Geographical habitat of the Baganda in Uganda
- Dhupadhola - spoken mother language of Jopadhola
- Google - Internet Search engine
- GP - General Practitioner only applied or referred to an appropriately qualified medical practitioner.
- IV - Intravenous - refers to a method of injecting food, blood, water, etc., into the body as appropriate.
- Jopadhola-nationality located in the Eastern part of Uganda, part of the wider Luo person
- Japadhola - describes the person identity arising from the being of Jopadhola.
- McDonald - Refers to takeaway eats, which originated in the USA but now is universal
- MOT - **M**inistry **o**f **T**ransport (United Kingdom) authority to validate that the vehicle is roadworthy.
- Muganda - describes a person of Ganda nationality.
- PhD - Doctor of Philosophy
- Scar - A mark left on the body after a wound or injury has healed.
- VIP - **V**ery **I**mportant **P**erson

Foreword

"...The pessimist complains about the wind; the optimist expects it to change; the realist adjusts the sails..." — William Arthur Ward (1921-1994)

I have known Jesse since the early 1990s when I first set foot on UK soil, on a postgraduate scholarship. Although I was living and studying up north, in the English Midlands, slightly over 100 miles away, I would come down to London once a month, at least, to meet up with friends with whom I was close while still back in Uganda.

Being among friends inevitably meant joining fellow Ugandans and, very often, fellow East Africans, in social gatherings to carouse and share the latest news from back home. Unlike today when the Ugandan community has become socially atomised beyond recognition, those were the good old days when Ugandans behaved as a tight-knit community, regardless of where they hailed from back in their homeland. Like plants in a dark cellar competing to catch an elusive ray of light, they looked out for each other as they struggled to strike root into the UK soil.

It was in such circumstances that I met Jesse and members of his immediate family, especially his indomitable older sibling, Flight Engineer Jack Alecho. We struck up a precious friendship that has endured all this long. Nothing special drew us together, initially; we were just Ugandans brought together through a shared destiny of being in a foreign land. In other words, our friendship evolved by osmosis. Otherwise, Jesse was - and still remains - an amiable giant with a sunny disposition always. On this particular point, I am yet to meet anyone who has breathed a bad word about him to me.

Thanks to the peerless ingenuity of Facebook, we discovered each other again for the first time in nearly 10 years of mutual silence. Nothing untoward had happened in the intervening period. Except what I characterised earlier as the social atomisation and rise of individualism in the Ugandan community in the UK. Those wild parties, nightclubs and political gatherings that were a defining feature of our unity as a people are all a distant memory now.

Against that backdrop, in this powerful memoir, Jesse is having a fireside chat – well, that is what it really is, just a chat, nothing else – with his immediate family, friends and workmates. But he has also some juicy bits for a diverse range of audiences: the general public, fellow Adhola people, professional colleagues, therapists, child development psychologists and, perhaps most important of all, life-course theorists. The bizarre thing about this memoir is that Jesse is more concerned about the hurt, pain and confusion his disclosures will have on the family, close friends, workmates and, surprisingly enough, even his own vicar.

You would have thought that any vicar worth his salt would be long accustomed to hearing tales of woe and despair from their parishioners. In a sense, you would be right. But not so Jesse; he is more concerned about how telling his vicar about his cancer diagnosis will affect him rather than how it is currently affecting him, this cunning patient-cum-purveyor of bad news!

Truth be told, I only first knew about the dreaded disease when Jesse contacted me in February 2020 and asked if I could give him feedback about a book he had written. I have long known from my keen interest in literature that all writers – especially budding writers - have an enormous need for someone to validate their work. Consequently, I was more than happy to oblige. And did!

I gave Jesse my new email address and he duly sent me his manuscript. I started reading and, into the first two pages, I stopped in my tracks. Why is it that it is cancer that has reunited me and my exceptional friend? I asked myself, not without a twinge of guilt. And as I write, that will be a difficult one to fathom.

So, when I gave him my first feedback, it was all I could do to blurt out that it was too emotive a subject to read with any measure comfort. Words had obviously failed me. I would be lying if I said I did not feel vulnerable and scared then. For lack of a better phrase, it all seemed like a fight-or-flight response. As I have come to expect, as soon as I expressed my deep feelings, Jesse threw a protective veil around me. He apologised profusely for the hurt and pain he imagined he had put me through by reading his manuscript. This made me even more confused and speechless.

I could not help thinking that Jesse was a figure of absolute fascination, an enigma. It is like knowing for the first time someone you have always known for a very long time. It feels and sounds like "*...We shall not cease from exploration...*" by celebrated American poet and essayist, TS Eliot (1888-1965).

Looking back, I know now that it was completely understandable for Jesse not to seek me out and share this grim piece of news. More remarkably, in this tell-all social media age, the news of his cancer diagnosis has not spread in the community, to-date. It is as if those who are privy to this are sworn to an omerta-like silence.

As far as Jesse is concerned, though, everyone and everything around him is *'mythical'*. Human nature is as much *'mythical'* as cancer is. Radiography machines and chemotherapy are all *'mythical'* - abstract concepts, if you will. None of these has a determinable basis of fact or natural explanation. This is one of those themes that Jesse keeps hammering home over and over again in this memoir.

A child development psychologist and a life-course theorist should also expect to discover how Jesse's childhood, boyhood and adulthood influences are helping him cope with his diagnosis.

Populating these stages of his development is a web upon web of social networks, a leaf venation that is his current life.

While he is gravely concerned about the emotional and psychological impact of disclosing his cancer diagnosis will have on people around him, at the same time, he very firmly recognises that it is they, more than anyone or anything else, who are providing him with extraordinary strength and resilience to stay alive and hopeful each waking day. And he is thankful to them all.

More to the point, all those influences have shaped his child-like - almost unserious - narrative in this memoir. Jesse is not angry with anybody. He is certainly not angry with God and, above all, he is not even angry with himself for living with a cancer diagnosis, nor does he wallow in self-pity. In this memoir, all he ever does is treat cancer like one of those vexing irritants; an unwelcome elephant in the room. He is, most assuredly, at peace with himself and with every constituent of his universe. Yes, he is fragile – we all are – but Jesse refuses to allow a cancer diagnosis to define his identity.

So, if you are expecting to read an angry book from a narrator who is wailing over the exigencies of a cancer patient's daily life; a patient wailing loudly over the gradual passing of a life well-lived, then you will be sorely disappointed. From my personal perspective, this is a narrative that may fill you with hope and power to thrive in the teeth of adversity. It is a cathartic roller-coaster. Every flower must grow through dirt. Don't you think?

Obalell Omoding
March 2020.

Introduction

The term 'introduction' has immense meanings. 'Introduction' is an art that has to be mastered. Therefore, in trying to 'introduce' you to the contents of this book, I have had to go through some serious reflective thinking. It's challenging to share a health-challenging journey by narrating it as a story, for it sometimes falls short of dramatising it as a sweet story to be read from beginning to the end. When a reader gets a book, it has to be interesting to read. One, therefore, ponders the serious health issue, in this case, 'cancer' associated with ending natural existence; would a person be interested in the narration of pain and suffering?

The mere mention of the word 'cancer' or to put softly, it is a ritual for this word to come out of the mouth the involved clinician, that is after slithering its way through the *'Mythical Tongue'* to reach the one affected. I guess the anxiety a clinician anticipates is such that an outcome/response is unpredictable. Just like in any outage, words have to be churned out before spitting them out to make sense to the listener, and to the reader, alike. This is all left to the *'mythical tongue'* to deliver that to the participant and or audience. Imagine the *'mythical tongue'* carrying such a load.

Now, having overcome that hurdle are follow-up hurdles of sharing the results of the clinical tests with loved ones, family and friends. Again, reactions of those near and far after hearing are just as unpredictable, more so the pains of telling and listening in unbearable. Next is sharing *'What is To Be Done?'* or *'What is Being Done?'* Whatever reference point that is being shared does not matter because 'what is heard from the one side of the ear escapes from the other, but the *'mythical tongue'* has done its work of delivery.

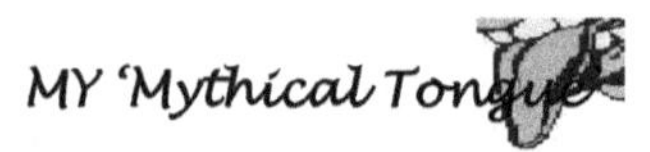

In short, it is the information no-one wants to retain. This is another ritual and the nearest I can associate is like being at the dentist to pull out rotten teeth. Here, I mean, there is the ritual for handling the anticipation of tooth-extraction, which is just as painful as sharing the next steps of doing the needful.

Now I had to pen this story or narration and can say it was hard, hard, and hard. To this end, I was helped by my brother Jack S Alecho, great-great-great-grandson of Oita, whose names you will find littered in this book as 'formally known as Seven-Thirty' and 'the Flight Engineer' who supported me in structuring all those rituals, anticipation, pains, etc., here as below. Obviously, and within reason, I have enclosed as much as possible the twists and turns of what I went through with 'cancer'. I have read about others who have been diagnosed with cancer. Each has a story to tell. It boils down to how to react, what to say or what not to say to them. Hence, for me, I have come to understand that I would give the same acknowledgement from whomever; for the disease itself is complex, so is the response to the giver or receiver. It means the reaction to cancer from the receiver, the ownership; no one description fits all types of reactions as it comes in all sizes. Hence:

An Open Letter To The Mythical Tongue

27/08/2018

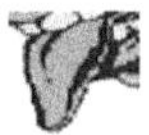

You are such a wonderful existence known and humanly placed inside the human race.

No wonder: -

> It is officially expressed as your tongue states where you come from!

Who you are! *Whom you are!* *What you are!*

How you are! *Where you are!* *When you are!*

Wherever you are! *Whatever you are!*

In other words, part of those differences is what is described as you having a *'Mother Tongue'*,

It may mean you belong to a certain category of people who speak similar to you.

It may help in differentiating you in terms of dialects.

It may mean that in some societies and cultures it can indeed tell from which 'class' you are born in or what you are trying to aspire to belong to or to be like.

You are well known in different spheres in a sense: -

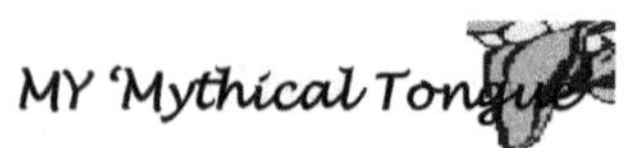

That you can wage a war. *That you can bring peace too.*

That you are mightier than a sword or a pen for other instances.

I have to believe in what is said about the *'mythical tongue'* because no one has a monopoly of the tongue,

I, therefore, respect it because the moment a tongue is identified with a mother then you know do not even go there; for a lethal weapon is around.

In me, you are my *'mythical king'*. The moment you are seething you forcibly antagonise the teeth to allow you out of the cage.

In response, the teeth also enforce the order; by ordering the mouth to open so that you can begin your utterance.

I am told you can be lethal but often you are also compliant.

You have such a powerful myth in you that often people fear what is going to come out of the twisted tongue;

Will it be a word? *Will it be words?*

Will it be a song? *Will it be ululating?*

Or will it be entangled words that you yourself may not make sense of at the time of saying it and is only reflected by others who hear it.

Why are you so powerful? I have come to learn over time that you are the king in me and that you can do anything. That is why you have to be *'mythically and safely guarded'* by both the upper and lower teeth and incorporating the mouth in the high-security fencing and gated not to allow you free will. You are known to be a *'mythical lethal weapon'* that can pounce anytime and at anything, as said by your confidants.

It may sound like you are in a prison, but actually, you are in paradise. I have seen kings', queens' and emperors' name them; are being tightly guarded and you rightly fit that bill.

In fact, a very close friend of mine who, for legal reasons I will not mention his name as he is a *bona fide* lawyer, once told me that if you want to keep it a secret don't say it even to your closest friend, like me. I had to ask him why? And he said anything out of your *'mythical tongue'* will come back to haunt you if you fail to discipline your *'mythical tongue'*. I wonder why he did not tell me to take every secret to my grave. But, anyway, if we happen to meet, I will ask him.

However, I learnt from then on not to let my *'mythical tongue'* wag-like-a-dog whenever I am aggrieved or feeling like saying something in haste; not to just say it just at the spur of the moment.

I remember when I had not learnt this art of not allowing my

'mythical tongue' a free-will gesture if I uttered the letter *'A'* someone would fill it with all sorts of letters of the alphabet from **A** to **Z** and sometimes it would even include numbers from zero to zillion. I would then sit back in a daze and lament how did the letter *'A'* from my *'mythical tongue'* warrant all these possible writs, explanations, expeditions and explorations,

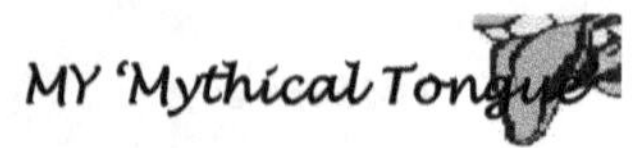

excommunicating of the whole of the universe to understand, justify and decipher the letter ***'A'***, honestly.

A tongue has both external and internal factors to deal with. It has to negotiate with the teeth to allow it to air its views and in turn, the teeth have to negotiate with the mouth to open up to allow the utterance of views the *'mythical tongue'* would like to express.

You can be amazed at how swift these negotiations can take effect and how fast the views are expressed, and the tongue goes back into hiding; as if it never said a word or did what others often say; *'said nothing'*. Such is the *'mythical tongue'*. The!! *'I never said that'* becomes the *'mythical rhyme'* and rhythmed by the *'mythical tongue'*.

Such is the precision and how dangerous the tongue can be. It is often said it can be lethal. The *'mythical tongue'* has no bones, but how it can launch such a vicious attack like a launched rocket and strong enough to pierce one's *'mythical inner soul'* and destroy it perplexes me.

In certain cultures, you find the tongue-twisting and just making noise, but that noise carries a thousand meanings and can be deduced to be very lethal, though often subtly done. Sometimes even pulling out your tongue is so condescending in certain cultures and can bring reprimand, so I hear.

Internally, the tongue has to make manoeuvres to ensure that anything palatable or unpalatable is tasted before churning it out to the rightful place. It has to agree with the brain that it is okay to say what it has to say. *'Mythical Tongue'*, it is funny when alcohol takes hold of the *'mythical human race'* remains an active participant, but the tongue takes the opposite. *'Mythically Slurred'* but thinks it is delivering what the human is thinking. In short, the body is alive, but the *'mythical tongue'* is in slumber and no collaboration whatsoever.

However, sometimes it delivers what the *'mythical psychic'* has been hiding for a long time and delivers the Dutch-courage, so I hear. The outcome can be as devastating as what the 'Dutch-courage' delivers often is not palatable.

The story goes: My *'mythical mother'* once bought a cow and named it *"Kirumi"*. I then asked her, what was in the name? That name was in Dhupadhola. That would literally mean *"does not end"*. She explained to me that the full meaning was that *"... to ..."* Basically, this means the person who utters a word easily forgets, but the hearer would never forget. Such is the power of the *'mythical tongue'* that it is capable of bringing out messages that can be received by another person differently and, meanwhile, you are moving on with your life, others have been hurt, destroyed or pleased along the way.

The *'mythical tongue'* is an inciting tool that can trigger peoples' emotions; it can set others to have an objective to fulfil the aims and objectives of others or self.

The *'mythical tongue'* can either be used usefully or uselessly. It has brought peace to others who use it diligently. It has also brought turmoil to others who use it recklessly. Used properly, the *'mythical tongue'* can bring harmony, freedom and this, in turn, can help growth and wisdom.

Sometimes I am one of these mythical goosey lots who think and think and does not allow my *'mythical tongue'* to do the outward somberness of uttering what I am mythically thinking. Sometimes, over time, I find myself trailing the trails. Sometimes it allows others to say what they think; I am meant to say or should say but in a distorted way. In reality, it has not been my *'mythical tongue'* that has said it, so I cannot own what others have tried to say as if it is on my behalf.

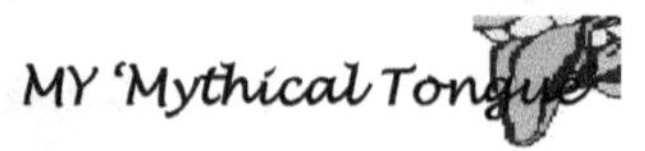

I learnt the art of denial while in a secondary school the hard way. That day and night, we were trying to set off a very dangerous situation while in my boarding school. I had a few friends and we went into this Bible and started quoting very dangerous quotes from the Book of Psalms. I tell you this book has very provocative words and can be used dangerously by various people to mean various things based on their own notion and understanding.

When the house prefects came to learn about it, they reported us to the housemaster-in-charge of our dorm, who called all of us. All my other friends were asked who did it and their *'mythical tongues'* were quick to say it was not them because that was not their handwriting. Their *'mythical tongue'* left me defenceless. I was left numb as I had used my skills to do the writing and my *'mythical tongue'* could not deny my own handwriting. My friends escaped and I ended up being punished for the sins my hands made to write what I and others had agreed on. Someone has taught me these words that: 'I died in the movie' on that day.

Since then I learnt my mythical lesson not to be dragged into a situation where *'mythical tongues'* will be wagging against me. Where my *'mythical tongue'* cannot authoritatively defend me, I keep my mythical mouth shut and not allow the *'mythical tongue'* to come out with teeth-gritting.

I have learnt that whenever my *'mythical tongue'* has to say anything it has to pretty have that private discussion, conversations, and consultations with all my bodily functions to check out whether it is feasible, palatable, and acceptable and within reason, for my *'mythical tongue'* to utter anything. Where there is doubt, my teeth and mouth would not open up for the *'mythical tongue'* to wagging like a dog.

So, just like other human species have their tongues, I have mine tongue too. I have honestly appreciated, over time, my *'mythical tongue'*; for its multi-tasking skills, such as food tasting, uttering words. Over time you have proved that you have mastered the *'mythical art'* in this weird world. I have learnt to listen to what you do, say, act, or decipher in my time of reminiscence. I have come to accept that you are mighty. You can help in tight situations to negotiate a way out or support in controlling the uncontrollable environment. I am also very much aware that you can be lethal either subtly or cunningly.

Often people think their *'mythical tongue'* owns all the knowledge in this world and have abilities that others do not have, and, have the sharpest *'mythical tongue'* as if no-one else owns one. In the end, things always catch up with them all because of their uncontrollable mischievous *'mythical tongue'*. Lastly, Humility is simplicity, or you can turn it the other way Simplicity is Humility. It is all in the *'mythical tongue'*, if well natured and utilised in the *'mythical tongue'*.

It has been confided in me that the *'mythical tongue'* often should as a matter of principle pass through three gates if it has to be believed. It is stated that it must pass the truth test, it has to pass the necessity test and the kindness test. I understand the failure of any of those three tests, the *'mythical tongue'* can be a lethal force.

However, sometimes on the spur of the moment, the *'mythical tongue'* can wag in an unfamiliar manner while assuming something is palatable and yet not. This then is taken in and the other organs begin to disagree with the *'mythical tongue'* choice of the day. In this instance, if it goes all wrong the tongue can be silenced for good and would never utter another word on this universe. Sometimes it is the other way round; the *'mythical tongue'* finds itself at the crossroad as it cannot no-longer utter anything because of failings in the coordinating subsystem in the internal organs. The *'mythical tongue'* then ceases to deliver messages, this leads to dangerous precedents unbeknown to the human race.

I have heard people say their loved ones never uttered their last words and often this has affected their lives or understanding why the *'mythical tongue'* never came up to say the *'mythical final farewell'* or word. I now understand that you do not sit there on the throne on your own, 'You' have to negotiate with others to bring out a meaning. When others are saying time is up. Time to go. It means Time is up/Shut shop/Move on.

The tongue liaises with various organs of the bodily functions and agrees on a strategy. That is why it plays such an important role and even being singled out and being used for identification purposes as my *'Mother Tongue'.* How *'mythical'* is that? It is purposely given the name for a reason. So is a *'mythical tongue'*, in the bodily function, a "She" I leave that for another day.

To be continued

JesseA

Pointers

As sub-headed, I capture four tenets, namely, Pain, Denials, Reflections and Outcomes; and the epilogue based on a timeline.

Chapter A captures the pain and learning from it. I have addressed this as it is often stated if you still feel pain it means you are still alive. Therefore, I can authoritatively say to you that I am still alive and can write and share with you my pains processes; for I can still feel pain.

Chapter B captures the denials and information management, as in all aspects of life we live in denial day in, day out. It is how we deal with those denials and channel our lives to a positive outcome if it allows you to open that door. Here, I recall all sorts of masks and camouflages in my cranium when I was challenged and struggling to fight and defeat this 'cancer'. Did I say *'fight' and 'defeat'?* Well, that was the thinking at every twist and turn and hence the heaving all sorts of shields and camouflage that saw me through the 'cancer'.

Chapter C captures the reflections and outcomes from all the pains, learning, denials and information management. It has helped me to unpack to you the journey I went through and outcome, if at all. Of course, in every journey, there is a learning curve. It is only through sharing this journey of mine that I can learn and support others in the journey too, whatever the journey. In the end, I can also support myself by continuously walking the path of the unknown. I have shared all these here because what appears or feels out of place may be the feelings that strengthened one, offered the resolve, however negative.

Epilogue captures the diary on the comings and goings before, during and the after the episodes as highlighted in the preceding Chapters. It has helped me unpack the factual journey and how that journey was navigated and who was involved across the swamps, lakes, oceans, seas and tortuous roads to deliver an outcome presented. I would say it is the healing part of the journey. Whatever you equate Healing to be. It is the realisation that whatever one goes through, there must be *'closure'*, however painful.

To be continued

JesseA

CHAPTER A

THE

P A I N

1.

An Open Letter To My Mythical Friend "Scar",

03/02/2018

Dear My Mythical Friend Scar,

Ever since I was born, it seems we have been *'mythical friends'* though I never knew you. I think to have always met you in all forms but always been invisible and sometimes *'mythically unreasonable'*. Well learned, naïve, friendly and genuine friends and families often tell me to get over it, such things happen in life, move on... Move on to where?

Over what?

Get over who?

Get over how?

Get over when?

Whose territory should I occupy when I have just lost mine *'mythical territory'*.

Asking me what is your *'mythical problem'*?

Okay, my *'mythical problem'* is the reason why you have been my *'mythical best friend'*. I don't have to *'mythically justify that'*.

I have met people to whom you are their *'mythical friends'* too, and they tell me to forgive you and forget you. So, true better said than done, but how can I leave you my best friend *'The mythical Scar'*.

Some tell me to turn to God in the heat or spur of the moment. I have often paused, reflected and internally asked myself this question; when was the last time; this person met and or held a conversation with God and I have not and how do they meet God the saviour?

My current *'mythical hallucination'* why is it not equated to having a conversation with God.

My *'mythical friend'*, you are such a thorn in the flesh; every time I see my healed wounds, I see your presence *'Mythical Scar'*. You even unmask my *'mythical scars'*.

Every time I lost someone you came all over me and created your presence. You have never left me alone, I wonder why?

You are always lurking in the back of all my *'mythical conversations'*. Even if I am *'mythically meditating'* in silence a tap on my shoulder assures me of your presence.

You have now made me understand your true self. I have had you in both visible and invisible *'mythical scars'*. You have such an attitude that you have now embedded yourself in my psyche. You are so notoriously notorious and sometimes too chaotically chaotic that I want to discard you, but then I question how that can be.

Do you remember what you did to me within the last year? You embedded yourself in me. I have tried to strike you off as my best friend on several occasions. You keep coming back to remind me to look at *'mythical this'*, look at *'mythical that'*, explore this, and explore that. And asking me is this *'mythically real'* or *'mythically fake'*. Indeed, they are all *'mythically real'* and you, my *'mythical friend'*; the *'mythical Scar'* is a part in *'mythical that'*! You keep coming back to me sometimes when I am low, you stoop low as well. When I am high you come stealthily also claiming the *'mythical moral high ground'*. Sometimes you come with these usual words at the end of a written letter **'Your Obedient and Faithful Servant'** as if you have *'mythical faith'* in me. 'You are indeed a *'mythical liar'*.

I have had numerous interactions, conversations about you, my *'mythical friend'' Scar'*. It seems so many people worship you because you are *'mythically real'*, you are *'mythically tangible'* and yet *'mythically aloof'*. Because you have created your presence in others' psyche, they address you in all forms, but the one fact remains you are a *"mythical 'Scar''*.

Okay, stop hiding and tell me why you don't only exist as my *'mythical friend'* but to all those, I have had contact with either face-to-face in any form or medium. You are a *'mythical scar'* to them too.

I have now come to understand that because you are called *'Scar'*, however, you are not *'mythically scarce'*, and neither are you *'mythically scary'*.

You seem to love me. You seem to understand me. Long after I last communicated to you and we had a candid chat, you again came knocking on my door. This time you knocked way high up the apex of my existence. You targeted my most inner *'mythical soul'*. You thought I could not see you, but I knew it was you. You had not gone away; you were still lingering within. You were testing my skills of guessing who you were/are, what you want and how you embed yourself in *'mythical vulnerable people'*.

You thought I couldn't see you. Well, you should have known this saying: *'once bitten, twice shy'*. But I never knew this phrase of once bitten, twice shy was your very *'mythical subject line'* that powers your *'mythical existence'*. So, you really knocked the twice shy person in me. You stealthily tried to walk behind my back but least knowing I had placed targets to get you Mr. *'Mythical Scar'*. Why do you think you can just walk into my life and do whatever you want to do and then walk away scot-free and unnoticed? As I stated earlier, you tried to use *'mythical scare tactics'* to penetrate your prey. You are such an obnoxious existence. If you have any human element in you, you care less about the repercussion. Now I know you have tried to create traps around to see how you can come stealthily and penetrate even where you are not supposed to be.

I will continue to safeguard myself against your nasty behaviour.

You are such an arrogant *'mythical twit in existence'* that you seem to think that you are the only *'mythical one'* who should *'mythically exist'*. That you are now like any other who is supposed to be around to create an aura to show that you are omnipresent, the invincible one and yet the devastating effect you leave behind is so inhumane for a lot to see.

Your behaviour is so *'mythically uncouth and diabolical'*; in fact, I loathe you – you disgust me - and please stop changing your colour like a *'mythical chameleon'*. You are not; you are just *'Mythical Scar'*. You need to own up to the devastation you leave behind. You need to think twice before knocking down the already the *'mythically vulnerable'*. You seem to think you are untouchable. Sorry, but I want to *'mythically loathe you'* and tell you straight in the face how I feel about you, right and simple you are *'mythical'* and *'mythically nasty'*.

To be continued

JesseA

2.

An Open Letter To My Mythical New-Found Friend Called 'Cee'.

25/09/2018

Hey, 'Cee'!!

On this day, the 25th of September 2017, you became part of me, you became my identifier; you became my form of identification. You became me and I became you. I walked into my GP's surgery for an appointment scheduled for 17:30 hours that day. I was called in, sat down and then asked to explain to the GP why I was there.

Prior to this appointment, I had a swallowing problem that I could not push in food unless I had a glass of water around me. If I forewent water by my side and pushed in food and it got stuck, I had to call for my son to get me water quickly as I was choking. That is when I knew I had to do something about it. That is when I knew I had to knock on my GP's door for assistance. I had now to accept that I needed facts and get out of the fantasy and fiction I was embedded in.

I wanted the GP to prescribe for me the right medication and not the type I was getting 'over the counter' as if what the one the GP was to prescribe for me, I would get either 'behind or under the counter.'

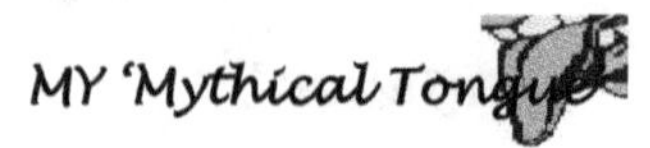

Alas!! I was wrong, wrong, wrong, wrong. The GP's computer said NO, No, No!!. The GP concentrated on his computer to type in information and with a bang, he had sent off the referral to hospital and out I was. Such are the assets of the computer-age, coupled with our own self-diagnosis.

I thought the GP would be this genius, but oh! no, it was not meant to be. I never received the prescription form to rush it to the pharmacy to get the right remedy. Instead, I was told to wait for a call from the hospital to attend for further investigation. The GP told me I should expect to wait for roughly a week for the hospital to call me and arrange an appointment to be seen.

He did not even bother or waste anytime pulling out his medical gadgets to examine me to know what was wrong so that he could sit back and hit his computer key for a prescription and send me off to the pharmacy to get a remedy. Oh No!! He did not do any of that! He did not even take a whisker instead he whisked me off to be examined and to be confirmed as a *'Cee'* patient.

I had never gone to a GP's surgery with an illness and walked out empty-handed but only being told to wait for another hospital appointment. I did not get any medication for relief. Such was the case of this ugly episode.

My GP, without as much as a glance, knew what was exactly wrong with me and what needed to be done. He referred me to the hospital where he knew I would receive some form of "hospitality". Days dragged by as my appointment for my first examination was to take place.

In my layman's mind, I knew there was something wrong as before this. In early July, I had severe chest pain and I got desperate of making a 999 call but somehow it eased out. That day was a Sunday; I had just come out of the church. That time I had a full package as there were a lot of things that had gone on and a lot of other things that were going on in my life.

From then on, I started going for over-the-counter medication to alleviate the discomfort I was experiencing. This, according to the medicinally qualified, call it "self-diagnosis" and medication. I thought in myself that I had developed possibly peptic ulcers. Hence, I tried to self-diagnose and I wanted to live within that picture, that sentiment and that belief that it would be manageable within my confines, within me and by me. Such are the denials that men build around themselves when faced with a vexing dilemma they do not want to address head-on.

Anyway, I had no option but to go along with the decision of the GP. I knew the situation was greater than what the GP could handle. Well, in this day and age of Google, googling, googled. I did just that. I typed in *'...Problem with swallowing and pushing food with water...'*, and bang!! I got a response from the boss 'Google'. The boss Google stated that: - *'...a possible common symptom of Esophageal 'Cee' is the problem swallowing...'*.

Immediately I shut down the system or was it my *'mythical system'* that *'mythically shut down'*? I never wanted to face the truth of what I had just seen and read. All along I suspected that my GP had diagnosed something along those lines but did not want to commit himself to tell me the plain truth.

Since the GP sent away my referral it lasted a week and phones started buzzing incessantly in the house and on my mobile trying to locate me. I got back to them as they wanted to talk to me so that they could arrange an appointment date for the hospital.

Never had I ever had an emergency hospital appointment like this referral. I was used to them only sending a letter with an appointment date and time, with clauses about non-attendance and striking you off. By contrast, this appointment was like thunder striking. I knew I was going to be in it for a long haul. We agreed on a date of the appointment, so it was for them to send

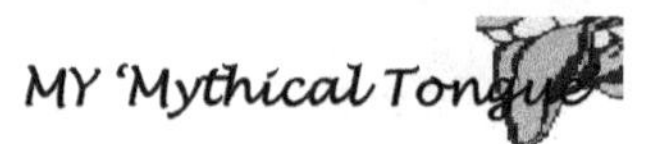

me a letter to confirm the date, time and place. Within a day I received a confirmation letter of the agreed appointment. It was a week on after this. I had to be prepared for that appointment to confirm exactly what boss Google had told me earlier of which I had closed my eyes to the reality of the truth.

As they say, 'truth hurts' and this is *'mythically true'*.

I had to go for an endoscopy to establish what the problem was.

Oh my! I started quivering at the mere mention of the word endoscopy as ten years earlier I went through a similar medical check and it was not a nice experience. I had to start liking that snake-like creature, snaking inside me as if looking for food, but actually looking for the diagnosis *per se*. This was going to be the Second Coming of this snake-tube going inside me. It was like "Aha!! You know what?" I should be that man who should stand tall.

You know what? *'Cee'*, you became an integral part of me. Apart and parcel of me. I had to begin developing a liking for you. I had to develop liking about you. I was, indeed, forced to develop a liking for you. In a nutshell, I had to be you. I could not get rid of you. However much I closed my eyes, you were there eyeing me; telling me porkies.

To be continued

JesseA

3

An Open Letter To My 'Mythical Snake Endoscopy'

28/09/2018

OH!! Mr Endoscopy

On the day of the endoscopy, I never went to work as the appointment was in the afternoon. I was prohibited from eating anything for at least eight hours. To me, because I had gone through the process before I knew that if I ate anything, the doctors would not work on me as when that snake goes in you when you have eaten you will throw up and the place would be messy. Therefore, I went on that day on an empty stomach.

When I arrived, I was welcomed, my blood pressure was checked, and it was high. The nurse asked me why my blood pressure was high. Was I thinking about the test? Obviously, I was anxious, and my blood pressure could not hide it - it refused to hide it.

I was then asked if I had come with anybody, which I understood to mean *'a companion'*. I said I hadn't and, anyway, in the letter there was no mention that coming with somebody was either a requirement or a necessity or even a suggestion. Anyways, I went in a body and that body was *'a mythical me'*. I was an adult, anyway, and capable of making own decisions whether I would require support or not.

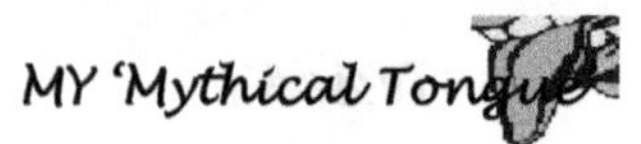

Shortly after that, I was given a bag to put in my belongings. I was then given a hospital gown and a wristband placed on my wrist that showed who I was and my date of birth.

When my turn came, I was given a detailed explanation of what they were going to do and getting me to sign a consent form for the procedure to begin. They numbed my throat and the process of pushing that gadget looking snake started its tortuous journey through my being.

To be continued

JesseA

JesseA's

Chapter B

THE D E N I A L S

4

An Open Letter To My 'Mythical Denial'.

18/05/2019

Hey!! 'Mythical Denials'

It was pinpointed to me that you are such a thorn in the flesh.

"Why d'you always come under the '*mythical cover*' that one doesn't know anything and in return you begin convincing me that, truthfully '*mythically*', I don't know anything and yet I do.

I found an expert in the field who looked at me in the eye and

asked me: "Why do you believe in the '*mythical denials*'. Why do you swear by denials in every '*mythical sentence*', every word every phrase you write or utter?"

The '*mythical expert*' had a go at me as to why I do not disown you and '*mythically expose*' you for what/who you are. That why do I hold everything to my '*mythical chest*' and fail '*mythically to explore*' the options of outing you in a '*mythical way*'? Out and out for everyone to see and feel whether you are worth or not worth me hiding you in my closet.

'*Mythical Denial*' hello!! You are such a compulsive liar! People can look you in the eye and see denials written all over you. So, why use me to hide you for others to see who you are and how worthless you actually are, really? You embed yourself in people and whisper into their ears to say, not to say it.

You *'mythically tongue'* twist people's tongues when they are about to say it and do a tongue twist so that they opt to keep silent and or lie.

'Mythical denial'; you are so demented that you want all those you have embedded yourself in to think like you!! You are not allowing people to say what they want to say, how they feel but they must look left and right in suspicion that what they might say may be given in evidence against them. Why the harassment? You try to create the court of law in yourself and want to be judge and advocate at the same time.

I was told you are so ingrained in people, especially those susceptible to *'mythical injuries'*, that they look for other options to camouflage those injuries and/or emotions.

However, I have to *'mythically learn'* that you are there for a reason in a season. You support people in their *'mythical fragile'* state to continue holding their *'mythical humanity'* without eroding of their *'mythical dignity'* and I respect you for that. For I have learnt that *'mythical dignity'* is such an important part of the *'mythical human race'* and it is you, *'mythical denial'*, who becomes the blanket cover for us and to hold us in order for us to have some *'mythical sanity'*. Thank you for being there on my *'mythical journey'*.

To be continued

JesseA

5

An Open Letter To My 'Mythical Anxiety',

16/05/2019

Hey! 'Mythical Anxiety',

I was asked by my *'mythical work colleague'* whether you do *'mythically exist'* inside me. I was asked about you when I was going for my review, one-year after treatment as to whether I was feeling anxious. It had not occurred to me that you would actually exist in a *'mythical way'* inside me. It was quite a bombshell that it was mentioned to me. Of course, I was taken aback.

On reflection, it was a boom!! You were actually very visible in me and I could notice you without a shadow of a doubt. You were standing in front of me and Intertwining yourself on me putting on some transparent invisible attire. I didn't know you are such a *'mythical pain'* in the arse!! Sorry mind my *'mythical language'*, but it is the *'mythical bitter truth'* that you actually *'mythically exist'* inside me. When I walked out of that door that day to get to my appointment the following day you became visible; you were moving like my shadow. You became my house keys, you became my mobile phone, and, actually, you *'mythically became'* me. You made me begin doubting own *'mythical self'* whether I had done this or had done that. Asking *'mythical myself'* where my keys are, where my phone is and yet are already in my '*mythical pocket*'. What a '*mythical cheek*'!!

You started making my '*mythical heart*' to '*mythically pump*' with '*mythical rhythm*', wondering what would be said to me the next day. Up and down my body you were encouraging the sweat to break out on me; imagine! You made my blood in me move at an unprecedented rate. I am not even sure whether I have that enough blood to meet your needs to go around at the rate you want it to move with vigour and at breakneck speed. What I will now call '*mine*' anxiety level hit the roof like. It was as if I was taking my car for a '*mythical MOT-check*' and thinking whether it would pass the one-year '*mythical MOT*' or fail and, therefore, require further repairs being done on possible dents or parts replacement, while thinking of the cost implications.

It had never crossed my mind that you are one of those things that create people's palpitations to rise. In fact, you are one of those things that ensure the heart ceases to function. If I may ask you, '*mythical anxiety*', why do you do that? Why don't you leave people alone to mind their own business? Why are you omnipresent in people? Why are you actually present in me? I don't understand your type of behaviour of visiting people without an appointment and going on clinging on to people as if you have nothing else to do and looking to do it on me.

In hindsight, maybe your '*mythical business*' is sourcing '*mythically unsuspecting people*' and actually to do it on people like me. Maybe your business credentials are to do on people like us who are unlikely to consent to work with you. Maybe that is how you earn your living by reporting of your achievements and I become part of your *'mythical statistics'* on your *'mythical spying'* on 'me' duties. But honestly, how do you do that? I am beginning to think the way you graft yourself in people like me and create that type of inference when the person has the least awareness is you actually; that is not amusing! It is damn wrong and if I knew your *'mythical superiors'*, I would report you to alternate superior powers, so that you are not only reprimanded for your antics but banished. Then who is me really!! I am just having a *'mythical hallucination'*.

If you believe you have true guts, you should present yourself in such a way that you can easily be recognised in public so that your attendance is acknowledged, and you get the true dose of your food. Rather than creating a cover and pretending you do not exist in people.

It is good that my colleague mentioned about you and now at any given opportunity. I check my health and it's you who make me check time and time and time again. You make me check whether I am really thinking right. You make me jump even when I should not jump.

You, *'Mythical Anxiety'*, do you also sometimes feel anxious that you may be caught out and be thrown out of your hidden drawer in people like me? You know what; *'Mythical Anxiety'*, that day when I entered the consultant's room my blood pressure might have hit the roof and now, I know it was because of you. Why did you do that? The moment I stepped out of the consulting room I felt deflated and started a different level of thoughts, whereby I had now to dash and begin informing others of the news from the consulting room. Were you still in me or at what time you had left and gone somewhere else? Or you became another *'Mythical Anxiety'*, who now was telling me to quickly tell others of the outcome. You can change faces like a chameleon. You are so fast in deciphering what is going on and how to change course.

You think you are clever; you think you are smart. I am sure there are smarter people out there looking for a rapid response invention which will counter your ballistic bombs to keep you at bay from people like me, you ensnare and encroach on them. You think you are the one who gives others adrenaline to think outside that box. But who tells you people want you to support them to think outside their boxes and yet you are the box who is outside? So, you want people to think and continue to *'mythically jump'* in your box that is *'mythically outside'* them. How many *'mythical boxes'* outside people's boxes do you have at a given time where you change from *'mythical hyper-aggressive'* to *'mythical dormant'*?

I wish they had just left you that name 'Anxious' it is also 'cool too'. So why did they add you this 'Anxiety' as if it is a Scottish name where they pre-fix *'Mc'* on *'Donald'* to become 'McDonald', and you the end-fix - *'iety'* - and remove the - *'iuos'* in it. What does that mean? I checked the dictionary and was informed - *'ious'* - is the end-fix. Yet when I searched in the dictionary for - *'iety'* that you end-fixed to your *'mythical name'* 'Anxiety', it does not exist. Why didn't you just leave it as Anxious then? That would be *'cool'* too and would make people to easily look you up and deal with you head-on. I now believe you are also a coward and Anxious as your own *'Mythical Anxiety'*.

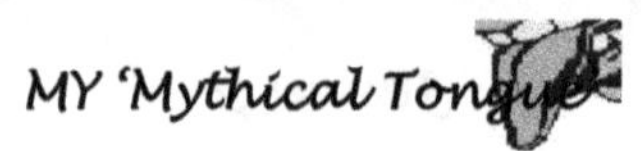

Anyway, to cut that long story short, there are now *'mythical lay people'* who can easily point you out as you were *'mythically pointed out'* to me by my very good *'mythical colleague'* and now I am aware that you like *'mythically hovering around'* people like me to ensure they continue being fragile, having low self-esteem, having self-doubt, so that you can thrive and report them to your bosses that you are heavily involved in doing wonderful work. I wonder how much you get paid every time you stick on people like a tick. I just Wonder!!

To be continued

JesseA

6

An Open Letter To My Mythical BNO

14/08/2019

Hey!! BNO

You know what! You have been the missing link from letter 'A' to 'O'. Having built up that *'mythical-chain-link'*, I feel complete and thanks for being there to hold the fort and to weather the storm.

You are that *'mythical hope'* that when I feel *'mythically down'* and out, I can shout, scream at and or cry on. You lift me up in my *'mythical dim circumstances'* and predicaments. You hold that *'mythical gate'* and strengthen the *'mythical bridges'* and I can cross without fear of falling over. What can I say? They say, say no more otherwise you spoil the soup. You have never spared the rod, nor have you spoilt the child.

You remember when you picked up that *'mythical call'* following on to my *'mythical anxiety'* discussion. You were quite concerned about my wellbeing. You know what? You were anxiety itself that day. We had quite a fruitful discussion and we rather came to agree. We joked and laughed about it but underneath there was a genuine concern and need to alleviate the pain.

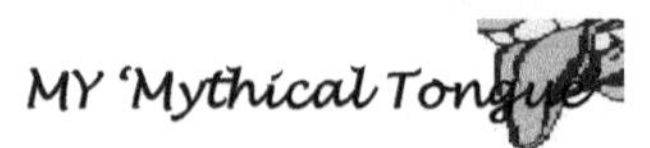

You remember when you gave me the prescription of the *'Mythical Aspirin'* this time around, I think you forgot that a year back you had prescribed similar *'mythical anecdote'* of prescriptions that I held dear throughout when you gave me the full dose. It carried me through then until other issues cropped up. I never looked away from your doses when you gave me; I kept taking them, swallowing them in prescribed doses. You know what? You are such a dispenser; how could you prescribe an aspirin the wonder drug *'mythically invented'* over 200 years ago and still going strong as if it was invented yesterday? You know the *'mythical aspirin'* prescription has had a *'mythical side effect'* in me. The side effect has done well on assurance and *'mythical cure effect'*.

Whenever I found myself in the *'mythical gutter'*, your *'mythical Aspirin'* prescription helped me get out of the *'mythical doldrums'*. It carried me along the *'mythical oceans'* of the unknown during difficult times and the *'mythical treacherous journey'* I went through. In a sense, whenever I came into some *'mythical dead-end'* - a *cul-de-sac'*, seeing no turning point, I could open the *'mythical dosage box'* and then kept taking it the way it was prescribed, the pains eased.

It helped me pull through; it never *'mythically disappointed me'* even an iota. Even a day when a meal could not get into me, your prescription became the meal. When *'mythical tears'* flowed down my cheeks and I wipe them off. I open your *'mythical dosage'* box and those *'mythical tears'* turned the tears of *'mythical pain'* to tears of *'mythical peace'*.

As I reproduce your *'mythical aspirin'* prescription below, you will *'mythically understand'* how you exactly cemented it where the heart is. Thank you for keeping on looking after *'mythical me'* and for me. You remember during our discussion when I sent you the note of prescription you thought was from a different physician. When I said it was from you, you could not believe it!! You know the same old saying; you can never forget your best teacher and I can never forget the best physician.

Sometimes I feel like getting *'mythically lost'*, but you keep poking me, pulling me out of my mire. I do not know how we came into this but by God's grace we are here; we are stuck to each other like *'mythical ticks'*. By the looks of it, I hit the *'mythical Gold'*. There have been so many things you have done behind my *'mythical back'* and only telling me when it was all over. You have watched over my back and have covered it so well. In fact, I can authoritatively say my back is fully covered and I am not complaining about it; for I hit a *'mythical jackpot'*.

> *"...He Has another Seed for You*
>
> *In Genesis[1], Eve went through great disappointment. Her son Cain killed her son Abel, the first murder in the Bible. I'm sure Eve, like any mother, was devastated and heartbroken at the passing of her son. But I love what Eve said in Biblical Genesis 4:25, "...God has appointed another seed for me...." In essence, she was saying, "...I don't understand it... It doesn't make sense, but I trust God... This is not the end... He has appointed another seed..."*
>
> *Friend, when you go through things that you don't understand, it is not the end. Nothing is lost in the kingdom. God is going to appoint another seed, and that*

[1] Biblical inference

seed represents the future. It indicates what is coming. If you will let go of what didn't work out, let go of the hurt and pain, then for everything you've lost, God will appoint another seed. You'll give birth to more in the future than you lost in the past. Keep praying, keep believing, keep hoping because God is for you. Trust Him and embrace the good things He has in store for your future!

A Prayer for Today

"Father God, You are the giver of all life! You give life to my dreams, life to my relationships, and life to my mortal body. Today I choose to release the past and embrace the gift of life you have in store for my future in Jesus' name. Amen."

Jesse, move on... Life continues, you have your life to live and take care of. We know the pain you are going through, but it is affecting your life - the life that Arnie and Kaio X R '01 *want around them to know that they have a father to protect them and love them.*

Stop looking behind and drive on. Your children want to see a happy and joyful Dad who will live and see their grandchildren".

Written and posted by My *'Mythical BNO'* on the 15/06/2017 via Hangout in Gmail.

To be continued

JesseA

7

An Open Letter To My Dearest 'Mythical Defence'.

26/08/2019

Hey!! *'Mythical Defence'*,

Why have you always lingered around me that you are defending me, claiming you are defending my rights, you are defending my existence and you are defending my very rights of the existence. Then why defend it; if it is mine and it had to help me in this journey.

The last time I heard about you was when you were mentioning the first line of defence is a *'mythical attack'*. Why create the first line of *'mythical defence'* when you should be at the forefront of that defence and not be in an attack mode? Why attack if the defence is your default option and mode? You seem to have allowed the first line of your defence on me to be the first line of attack. You allowed entries of all sorts of things to attack me, to disable me, jump into my *'mythical bloodstream'* to destroy me then you turn around and say you are defending me. Really, how defensive are you on applying the defence mode?

You begin holding me at ransom, yet you allowed my body to be attacked and wasted away. How are you like in the real *'mythical sense'* that you are a *'mythical defender'*? Hey, *'mythical*

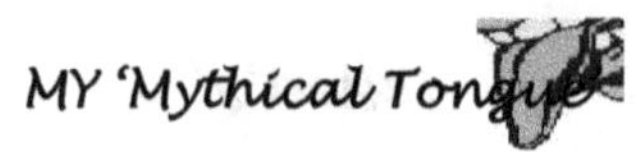

Defence'! You are really a defender of what? A defender of your own weakness or your wickedness? A *'mythical defender'* of allowing others to attack me what a defender who brags of defending yet allows every Jack and Jill[2] to access my body and do whatever they want to do then you turn round that you are defending me.

Hello!! Do you think we are *'mythical spring chicken'* who doesn't know how you operate? Get a *'mythical life'*! We know all about you that at the end of the day you are trying to do a job you are meant to do of defending though you are also defenceless.

Sometimes you act *'mythically crazy'* with your defensive mechanism that has no *'mythical mechanics'* in it. Where did you learn the *'mythical art of defending'* to begin articulating yourself that you are a defender? Maybe I would suggest you do a deed poll and change that name as I have not seen anything in you worth holding on as my *'mythical defender'*.

Then again, sometimes you may have, after all, defended me in my time when I least expected; I would get out through that eye of a needle and could not explain how. To me, that is a phenomenon and it might be down to you, my omnipresent. In that sense, I have seen your greatness in behind the scene defending me to avoid going into the unknown. You have defended me to keep me afloat in the times and the periods when I didn't know the 'ins' the 'outs' the inside and the whatever. Here I am now also defending your rights of existence. You scratch my *'mythical back'* I scratch yours the story goes on and on.

When I was young, we used to think because our grandfather was old, we could do mischief, runoff and we would not be caught and disciplined. My *'mythical grandfather'* whom we called 'Ofano' short for Stefano had his motto. *"Iringo t'Awotho"* - Meaning *"You run... I will walk"*. Whenever we did anything wrong when he stood up with his walking stick, we took off while he would walk

---

2 http://www.wordsforlife.org.uk/songs/jack-and-jill-went-hill

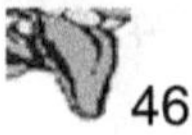

slowly, and we could run very fast. Stefano's first line of defence was the *'mythical high grass'* that surrounded the homestead, that we could not run into. His next line of defence was the *'mythical massive forest'* we had that we feared to move into so you would become disabled and just simply give in.

So, Stefano's motto taught me that I may be a very *'mythical fast runner'*; he always had the last *'mythical laugh'* for what he had was the line of defence and he knew damn well how to defend his '*mythical territories*'.

To be continued

JesseA

8

An Open Letter To My 'Mythical Sin'.

15/07/2019

Hey!! My Mythical ***s'I'n***,

I often go to church and hear *'mythical sermons'* whereby the words *'mythical'* 'I have sinned against you' are so much ingrained in the prayers. I have often wondered why we say I have sinned and do not mention the sins committed. It might mean it is quietly mentioned internally without externalising it.

I have done my own *'mythical soul-searching'* around my *'mythical sins'*. I commit per second of every time I breathe in and out. In the midst of all this, there is this bang! Sin! Three-lettered words and between these three letters lies this notorious *'I'*, meaning me, *I* and myself.

Each time I mention the word 'Sin' it points at me. It means it is always *'I'* in the sin so nobody else commits that sin apart from *'I'*. Therefore, sin cannot be a collective thing as it is only an *'I'* thing.

It dawns on me that the *'mythical sins'* that I committed per second are the sins I request to be *'mythically forgiven'* for, because *'I'* sits comfortably in the sin. In essence, it means it is all about those things that I hold dear in me and cannot share it outwardly with anybody else. Otherwise, if I share it out with anyone, anybody, everybody, it ceases to be sin for I stop owning the; *'I'* in the *'mythical sin'*.

I have come to dissect and understand that *'mythical sin'* is a daily occurrence and requires daily *'mythical forgiveness'* for they are the *'mythical things'* deep close to one's *'mythical heart'* that may be *'mythically painful'*, done or undone and cannot be shared with anyone even within myself for it is that secret and internalised in our *'mythical inherited psyche'*.

Anything shared or mentioned ceases to be a *'mythical sin'* for you have shared it externally in the *'mythical public domain'*. It cannot be forgiven in *'The Sinning against You'* mode of *'I'*. It, therefore, means my *'mythical sin'* is personally mine till the end I will ask daily for that forgiveness wherever that opportunity arises. For sin is sacred; once I have sought that forgiveness, I become whole or holy again, the slate is clean done and dusted. I am aware that once I have asked for the forgiveness of my sins in the *'I'*, then, I have no more guilt in it as I no longer own it.

However, if at any point I disclose whatever I have classified in the *'mythical sin forgiveness'*, then it ceases to be a *'mythical sin'* as it comes out as a *'mythical by-product'*, you may call it *'mythical puke'* if you wish for it is no longer the, an *'I'* thing.

To be continued

JesseA

9

An Open Letter To The 'Mythical RMH' Institute Of Excellence[3].

18/03/2018

Hey!! *'Mythical RMH'* Institute of Excellence

You were such a brilliant *'mythical lot'*, you taught me how to *'mythically fly'* within your *'mythical simulator'*. The first day I was *'mythically introduced'* it was in the *'mythical Hawthorn Simulator'*. You made me feel at ease during the time I was *'mythically inducted'* how to *'mythically fly'*.

I was introduced to the *'mythical first session'* that was to last up to *'mythical 30 sessions'* of simulator *'mythical training'*. What a well-dressed RN! You were such fantastic professionals; your work was *'mythically flawless'*. I wondered that when introduced and when I asked questions *'mythical information'* answers just *'mythically flowed'*.

You have *'mythical seven simulator training areas'*. Hawthorn where I had my basic training then subsequently transferred for the long training duration for the course duration at Rowan, and once I enjoyed Juniper when my session at Rowan due to the servicing of the machinery. I *'mythically enjoyed Juniper'*.

---

[3] https://www.royalmarsden.nhs.uk/royal-marsden-school

I used to wear *'mythical worries'* up my *'mythical forehead'* and up my *'mythical sleeve'*. It was a *'mythical method'* to show the *'mythical others'* who would be the *'mythical highest bidder'* to take out or over these *'mythical worries'* and *'mythically own them'*. Over time, I have learnt not to put my worries up my shelves for shoppers to come and buy and/or snob. By doing so, I now own my own worries, I no longer look for *'mythical shoppers'*, for I realised that I am not the only one in this *'mythical world'* who has *'mythical problems'* and/or issues.

Other *'mythical simulators'* were Beech, Willow, Mullard and Cedar. I was *'mythically told'* that on average *'mythical 30'* ***'Cee' students*** were seen per day per simulator. Imagine *'mythical 30'* ***'Cee' students*** per day x 5 days per week per simulator across *'mythical 7 simulators'*. It means on a rolling monthly a lot of *'mythical* ***'Cee' student's*** graduate from the RMH institute of excellence.

This shows you a glimpse of how many *'mythical* ***'Cee' students'*** within the institute catchment area attend sessions and graduate after that.

It shows how busy the *'mythical* ***'Cee' students'*** training Centre is and how good the faculties are. I was impressed and also overwhelmed that those who graduate must be many you know!

One time someone told me if you want to know that you do not have any problems you go to the hospital and you will realise how your problems are a very tiny fraction of those others who cannot advocate for themselves, who cannot get out of their hospital beds to help themselves.

I used to think that life moves in a *'mythical straight-line'* where there were no *'mythical junctions'*, no *'mythical bends'* but it was like a beaming light that travels in a straight line. Over time, I have come to realise that life is a *'mythical journey'* full of ups and downs, full of potholes, full of success and failures, full of junctions, full of everything just mention them, they are all '*mythically true*'.

I was booked into '*mythical RMH*' for medical assessment and that is where I realised that there is an illness, and there's 'is' '*mythical illness*' too.

I realised illness does not '*mythically discriminate*' based on race, culture, age, abilities name them.

The one thing that I wanted to say was to RMH, I give my '*mythical thumbs up*' as it is a hospital purely for 'Cee' clients and I tell you the gadgets available are quite exquisitely amazing.

The names of the radiotherapy treatments room quite unique as it gave the understanding that these '*mythical human radiotherapy simulators*' were quite advanced. There were the '*mythical Beech, Rowan, Juniper, Willow, Cedar, Hawthorn, and Mullard*'. It so happened that I was '*mythically schooled*' in Hawthorn, Juniper but I was more '*mythically enrolled*' in the Rowan that also happened to be the children's machines as they were being wheeled each morning from their wards to come for the therapy. Those are one of the things that were touching to me to see infants too were not spared of this illness and put my thumbs up to the medical fraternity for all the works they do. I have remained and been humbled by the nature of dedicated team working in that environment where you are literary trying to redeem sometimes a lost cause, but they still try against all odds.

To be continued

JesseA

10

An Open Letter To My Dearest 'Mythical Negativity Effects In Me'.

01/04/2019

Hey!!'Mythical Negativity Effects In Me'.

The day I realised that disengaging the *'mythical negative terminal'* to complete a *'mythical circuit'* was itself *'mythically positive'*. This was the day I realised that negativity was just *'mythically redundant'*, and *mythical* positivity was the *'mythical buzzword'*. For how long have we *'mythically been peddled lies'* that positive and negative completes a circuit, but negates the positive, hence rendering it *'mythically ineffective'*?

By disengaging the *'mythical negative polarity'* out of the circuit, it brought the *'mythical serenity'* in me. It created that *'mythical alkalinity'* in me and every aspect of the *'mythical acidic deposit'* that was being *'mythically deposited'* due to the two *'mythical circuits'* coming in contact and corroding the system had to be *'mythically scraped off'*.

It delivered that *'mythical ultimate touch'* of *'mythical positivity'* within the *'mythical serenity'* of disengaging the negativity. It rendered the very *'mythical soul'* of my *'mythical existence positive'* with an alkaline touch. By so doing the disengagement it enhanced my *'mythical wellbeing'*.

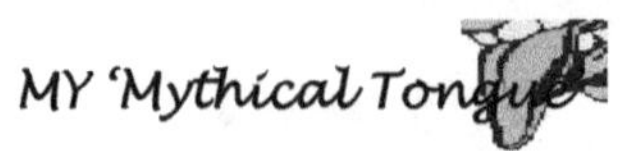

It brought that inner *'mythical sanity'* in me to reflect all the *'mythical dirt negativity'* deposited on my *'mythical positive terminal'*. It made me clench my *'mythical fist'* that at last a *'mythical bulb'* could be lit without a *'mythical circuit existence' 'mythically completed'*. Who tells you there are only the *'mythical scientific models'* to every *'mythical scientific problem'?* There are also the *'mythical social models'* that play in that, but it requires an art to do it and not the *'mythical science'*. In the end, it lit the light for my own wellbeing. It showed that even in that deep darkness there is light. There is wisdom and there is *'mythical tranquillity'*.

Alas, why couldn't I think of this long time ago to have experimented on this *'mythical scientific model'*? Well, life changes help build the *'mythical mind'* to reflect on things that threaten your own *'mythical existence'* too much of *'mythical negativity deposit'*.

To be continued

JesseA

Chapter C

REFLECTION AND OUTCOMES

11

An Open Letter To The 'Mythical Antics With My Grandfather'

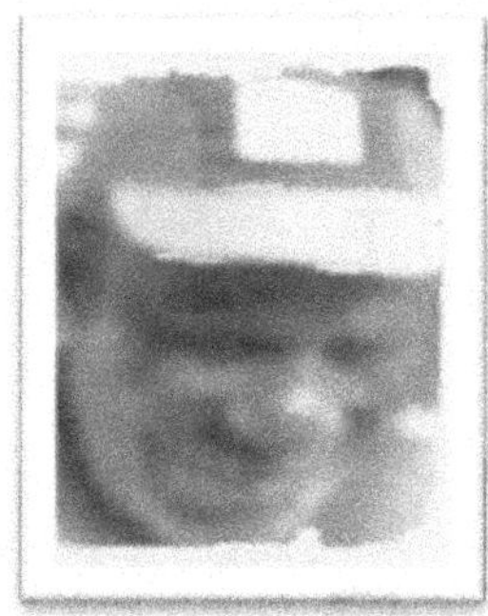

30/08/2005

Hey!! Mythical Antics With My Grandfather'

I want to share with you a little adventure while under the umbrella of my namesake, my grandfather (Grandpa). In the youthful days, Grandpa offered me some good lessons and practice guide how to sense whether White Ants *[agoro/ripo /sisi/ miyali/ olumbe/ magere]* is about to be harvested or not. I will mainly dwell on the *"Agoro and Ripo"* as they are mostly harvested at night. Grandpa trained me on how to perfect the art of White Ants' harvest. The rainy season normally accompanies White Ants harvest period. The bushes are fully grown and green.

On the day/night White Ants are anticipated it should normally rain as a principal rule. The dew is left hanging on the bushes ready to take you through the rituals. I had to learn how to avoid being drenched by the hanging dew, by skilfully dodging the over and undergrowth along the thin winding paths, Grandpa and I travelled to and from the Anthills.

Grandpa taught me how to build a tent-like cover using green banana leaves on the anthills to make sure we got the maximum White Ants [*Agoro*], for a season's feast. As some or most of you may be aware, getting and harvesting White Ants is a tedious business. It involves staying awake for the night to make sure that the monitoring process is thorough, and the White Ants would actually make your night, that night. It involves timing when to cover the anthill, for it to gain the desired warmth and enough drizzly rain for the termites to break loose the aperture the cheeriest White Ants are to come from.

The timing as to when to check that the White Ants are about to come out was very crucial. For the case of White Ants, it comes out respective Anthills at about 1 to 2 am. By around midnight we would normally check that the Anthill had gained warmth. The next thing we had to check was that during this time we had to understand the type of termites moving around the aperture. This was always done by pushing a lemongrass or spear-grass into a hole. If only big termites held on to the lemongrass, we normally kissed White Ants collection goodbye for that night or maybe even for that season. However, if some big ones were mixed the small ones at the further end clinging on the Lemongrass, a harvest was assured. This would confirm to us that we were about to get that year's harvest. If only big ones were clinging on the Lemongrass, we easily gave up and folded up to later end of night's sleep.

On one occasion I got the standard diagnosis, everything looked so positive that the harvest would be ours. However, forty winks weighed heavily on me. I deluded my grandfather; we all folded up to have forty winks and at the daybreak alas! White Ants' feathers were all over. I still do not want to share the experience I received for this fallacy as it is, still feeling raw on my nerves.

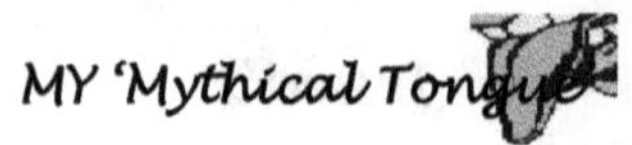

However, I have only taken the positives and to-date, I eulogise Grandpa even in his everlasting sleep. For he taught me the antics of knowing when the fruit of labour is near and whether it could materialise. I learnt from Grandpa when to have my forty winks but not through fallacy.

To be continued

JesseA

12

An Open Letter To My Mythical Grandmother Tolo

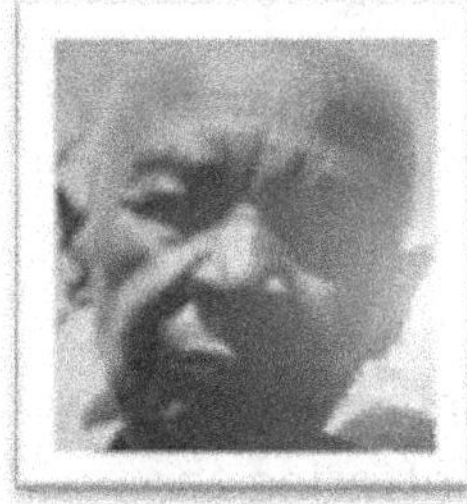

15/08/2018

Dear My Mythical Grandmother Tolo,

My Dear Gran Tolo (Grandma), hello long time no see. My Grandma was such a disciplinarian. You would not pass her clinician discipline. Yet she was often fair. When she knew you were remorseful, she would do a laugh with dimples around her two cheeks, showing you her distinctively open middle gap in the upper teeth.

The one thing I remember her for was her teaching process that often she said;

> *"you could have all the education in this world but if you did not have the 'Komi Gi 'Kiseke'; meaning in her tongue-in-cheek "commonsense" then no matter what you would do in life, you always would falter".*

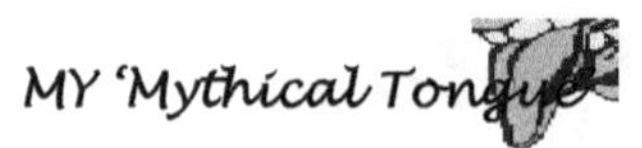

Tolo you will love to hear this wherever you are now there is the *'mythical intellectual'*, one of the first graduant of the Tolo University. He reflected to me the meaning of your *'Komi Gi Kiseke'* he challenged my *'mythical notion'* expressed by letting/taking me through the *'mythical ancestral libation'* that he quietly acquired during his *'mythical visits'* when he was called to acquire the *'mythical stool'*. He told me that the *'mythical traditional' 'Komi Gi Kiseke'* in Tolo's university *'mythical syllabus'* included her taking you through the *'mythical rituals'* of understanding the concept model of dealing with ordinary day-to-day activities that included, very common things such as receiving a guest upon arrival in the courtyard - She would *'mythically whisper'* in your *'mythical ears' 'weyi mi'ngo''* [meaning stop your stupidity]. As a young person, you welcomed the guest and the first thing you provided the guest was the *'Komi'* [chair] before offering the guest *'Kiseke'* [straw] that would include a drinking water. He told me you would fail the Tolo University *'mythical entrance test'* - if you provided the guest with *'Kiseke'* first before *'Komi'*. It would show how unlearned you are - She would *'mythically compound'* that *'neni me paka i'ming'* [meaning see this one is very stupid]; by giving the guest *'Kiseke'* [straw] before *'Komi'* [chair], hence my *'mythical 'common sense''* area of explanation filling the gap.

I remember in her lifelong learning *'mythical school'* she taught the art of winnowing. Oh my!! Grandma was a *'mythical PhD'* itself in that. Her winnowing tactics were with precision. When she was lecturing the art of winnowing millet using the traditional winnowing tray, the concepts were different from winnowing groundnuts, peas or any other stuff. It was like going to the University and finding various departments of science, social science, engineering, name them, but she was the only main head of all those departments. Call it dictatorial, dictatorship, dictator, whatever she was the one and only.

Grandma's winnowing tray was always prepared first thing in the morning, she would tell you to fetch cow-dung and then she would ensure it was smoothly smeared both inside and outside and then dried out under the sun. She would ensure when the winnowing tray was dry, she would wipe off any protruding dried dung left. Then her schooling would start.

If it was a day for winnowing millet, she would ensure that the millet was got from the granary and dried under the sun. Then, depending on the quantity, it would either be pounded using mortar and pestle or put in the courtyard, then using nicely prepared logs were used to hit it until that millet saw the sense of the day.

Grandma's first stage was to ensure that as the millet was getting out of the husks, she would start with the seeds that had come out first. This is where you would see her expertise get the better of that millet. As I stated earlier, winnowing is an art. It is not scientific, it is not arithmetic, either! If you did not pass through this school, you would falter.

There was a way she held the winnowing tray in both hands as she kept on shaking it to remove the pure seeds from the chaff and then would in a split-second winnow of the chaff in a blink of an eye. She would then continue this process until the seeds were left bare.

However, to remove the '*mythical useless seeds*' that would not make good millet flour, she would then churn the winnowing tray around and in a split second or two, the unneeded seeds would see the end of the day out of the winnowing tray on to the ground. It was then left for the perfect millet seeds to tussle it out with any stones, or sand that would spoil the eating of millet.

This Grandma would go on and on and on, slowly but surely, by churning and winnowing it left into right until the sand/stones

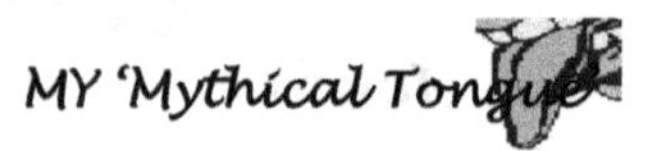

began sitting on her right-hand side of the winnowing tray. She would then, in a matter of split seconds, twist and turn the winnowing tray into both hands. Then it would be the left hand that is left to hold the winnowing tray in that split second as the right-hand captures the now visible sand or stones catapulted into the air and is discarded.

That is when I knew that the art of winnowing required *Komi gi'kiseke* [commonsense] and the need to have those tough training. As a boy growing up I had to learn the art of winnowing and this during this time, helped me shape my brains just as I used to see my Grandma churning, twisting the winnowing tray left into right into right and left and retaining the actual millet needed for food and discarding the chaff, stones, and sand into the oblivion. Over time, it developed my brain to brew, ferment and distil her principles of articulating the winnowing model into other concepts of thinking.

I found out that this winnowing model could help in winnowing off in your brain the chaff from the millet and the stones, sand from the seeds that you required to make good food. This sharpened my brains into hearing from so many people, especially those who may have passed through this type of education my grandmother gave to be swearing that I would only eat the millet that has come from my mother. Implying that commonsense prevailed in ensuring that what is going to be put on a plate deserves the attention/precision like my grandma's Tolo-teaching University, from which the many benefited.

I have also been at long last been a privy from our *'mythical Commander'* that mbu! You classed them how to bring up children straight and narrow. That she learnt that from you, of course, it seems also that she may have got that commandership model from you as she confided in me that you used to escort them to school and ensure they have attended the classes before walking home.

That they also now remember the good Cow Ghee [*Moo Dhiang*] put in *Magiira* [split peas] and using three-fingered cassava stem to whisk it to be smooth and eaten as a sauce. She told me that she enjoyed that and respects you for passing via your University. You may have spat saliva on her right hand to take over your charms. My understanding is that is how traditionally elders pass on certain traits and inheritance. I wonder if she can also go into the bush and brings out those traditional herbs to cure illnesses the way you used to do.

Who would argue with that? Tolofaina deserves a medal especially to those who passed through her school and have also taught others what she taught them. I stand to be counted among the graduands of her school of winnowing lectures. If you have not passed through that school you could be hoodwinked by the time you realise you have been winnowed out into oblivion and eating stoned, sand infested millet. That is why I love you Tolo. Long live your Tolo-University training in the art of winnowing.

To be continued

JesseA

13.

An Open Letter To My Mythical Dad IOA.

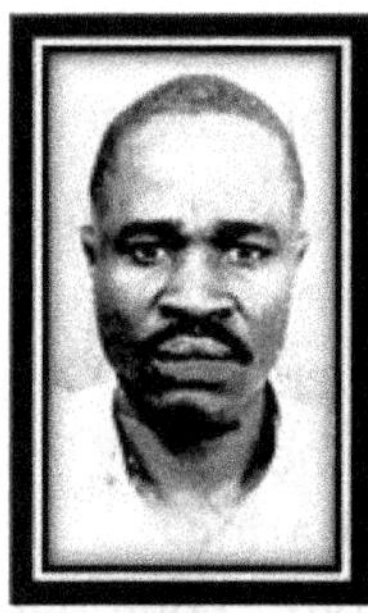

10/08/2018

Dear My Mythical Dad IOA

Whenever I listen to this song by Labi Siffre[4], '*...Something inside so strong, I know I can make it...*' it gives me that '*mythical reflection*' of how your presence is still '*mythically omnipotent*' though departed 60 years ago.

I have been fed these '*mythical stories*' about you and your ambitions over time and have quite often met people who years down the line when they met you and an introduction, they accord

4 https://www.google.com/search?q=labi+siffre+so+strong+lyrics&rlz=1C1GCEA_enGB852GB852&oq=Labi+Siffre&aqs=chrome.2.0l6.4405j0j4&sourceid=chrome&ie=UTF-8

you respect as if you are still present. They say how you changed their lives; I wonder how.

In this world you thought you were the master mastery of things at a tender age you graduated into teaching became headmaster, became an inspector of schools, become a District Councilor and even wanted to share/support in carrying the mantelpiece of Uganda's independence.

I am wondering how you managed to achieve all these things in a short while. In today's Uganda, it would be deemed you were corrupt or there was nepotism taking effect. But you were in the terrain of colonial times where everything had to be perfect in Africa Speak.

I am told you bought land in Siwa, Mulanda county, then wanted to buy land in Osukuru county. If my memory serves me well, you had land in Loka'omwa and the one we settled in. In Lwala to-date it has not been tampered with. What I saw was a white Ford Escort that you acquired prior to your death.

My remembrance is you had land in Loka'omwa that one I saw, and the one we settled in, in Lwala P'Obona village to-date it has not been tampered with. Another tangible thing I saw was a white Ford Escort box-body that you acquired prior to your death.

I was privy to a conversation that you were maybe the first Japadhola to have allowed your wife, then aged 25 yrs old, to get out of the kitchen and deal with the public good, hence you taught her how to drive and take control. This earshot conversation was being aired out by none other than a Japadhola, a traversed Doctor, who has moved all over Africa dealing with complex medical issues known to the human race. He is none other than the '*mythical Dr O'Ojony*' of '*mythical Pajwenda City*'. This has made me look at you in a different light than what others have previously

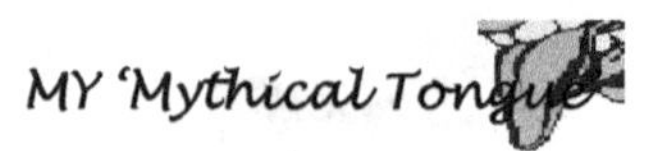

told me about your openness and abilities to embrace new cultural norms at that age and in the analogue era.

It seems you wanted to build an empire and safety- net for your family, but your life was cut short at a tender age of 36 years. You left us in a forest of untapped resources, a mud wattle house with the corrugated iron-sheets roofing. My mother, who was your wife, told me that the day we moved from Mbale Town to Lwala P'Obona village when the lorry carrying our household tearing through the spear- grass to reach the new home and left us in that forested place. She told me, that I started to cry running away from this wild homestead that I wanted to go back to Mbale Town chasing the lorry. What an irony shortly you left us in that vast untapped land and went back to your ancestors, the Creator.

As narrated by your wife that you left being an Inspector of Schools and instead opted to come back to Nabuyoga Primary School to teach, that allowed you to become a District Councillor. You were representing Bukedi District at Maluku, in Mbale Town, together with '*mythical Balaki Kirya*' [RIP], from Bugwere, '*mythical Yakobo Maloba*' [RIP], from Samia, and '*mythical Joseph Washukulu*' [RIP] from Bunyole. From this '*mythical Maluku*' place is where your journey started to '*mythical Entebbe Town*' and hence your demise.

A close family friend gave me an insight upon your death. There was the that further enlightened me about this '*mythical aspect*' that in our culture you cannot die without being bewitched *[translated in Dhopadhola that Dhano ki'tho mu'ngoye jajwoki]*. In Sweden I met our '*Mythical Owuya*' and we had a lengthy chat and discussion a night away about you and his late dad, Mr Opoya Ragang. He gave me an insight into how upon your death the fingers were pointing to the Catholic faith that they were the ones who had bewitched you. So, there was a general clarion call that no Catholic should come to your funeral.

However, his dad, the Late Opoya Ragang defied the call and told them that you were his friend; he saw no religious bias. You were a fellow teacher who was advancing the education in Padhola and saw no reason why he should boycott your funeral. He came and did his ritual, and nothing happened, the story goes.

All over Padhola: On reflection of what my *'mythical Owuya'* confided in me, I now had a mind gaping thought that no wonder, it became simple for our family became amongst the first to have been enrolled in a catholic school in Siwa as a protestant family, where Opoya Ragang was a teacher there. He was instrumental in ensuring that we felt safe, secure and where never bullied, as being of a protestant family. In a nutshell, such is your intertwined legacy.

Allover padhola if you are introduced as coming from *'Isirayiri's* family is like there is only one *'Isirayiri'* in padhola, people will accord you all the due respect. So, here I am reliving your praise while on earth however short your life was. To date I am still Isirayiri's child, imagine that. It made sense to a lot of people. A life journey is not about how long you live on earth but how much you have touched people's inner soul and made a difference in their lives however minute. You are the story being well told, I wish you were here, but I know you are listening and also recording. I have been privy to your *'mythical listening skills'* and I am very aware you are taking note and will communicate when the time is right.

To be continued

JesseA

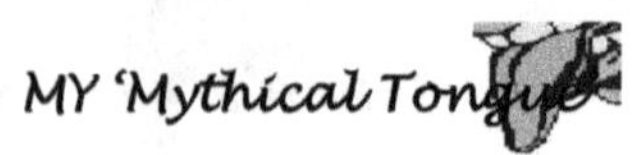

14.

An Open Letter To My Mythical Paternal Grandparents Ofano And Tolo.

13/08/2018

Dear My Mythical Paternal Grandparents Ofano And Tolo.

I have had to shorten the names because it sounded 'sweet' then and still sounds 'cool' now. Their names in full are actually Stefano and Tolofaina. I have loved my grannies to every bit of an inch or millimetres of their lives on earth while intertwined with own life while hoovering over this earth. It was such a blessing to have had you as my grandparents. It indeed showed who you were during your own reign on earth.

You never faltered an iota. In fact, you proved to the world -over though others may not know that you stood above parochial thinking or mindset and delivered the impossible to be possible. You made what looked like a mountain to be an anti-hill.

You were such great guys ahead of your time. I have been wondering how to articulate myself having brought us to earth and be what we are today though others have since followed you to that resting place. However, I have to give up my personal space, as I do not want to overcrowd my space with others who may not have my or similar thought process.

I would like to take this angled approach to my appreciation how you have shaped my thinking to look at my own life through the prism of your lenses and transformation of how you delivered me to be what I am today.

I am therefore writing to both of you this Open Letter to appreciate the sacrifices you made for my own existence and growth, on this earth. You are such an amazing couple I am proud of you to call my grandparents [my father's parents].

I wish to start on a reference point of your greatness; is the point of your own sacrifices as a couple. I have never known any better couple than the two of you.

You two invested in your eldest son to become a-somebody in order to fill up the gaps that the two of you never had the chance to. You offered it all, so I am told. You made efforts sacrifices to make him a-somebody. Because you educated him, he became employable. You showed him that marriage is the way to offer and build a family. He did just that and passed it with a tick including a church wedding. You gave him the inclination that in marriage children become the anchor of your existence. He was blessed with your grandchildren, all blessed and baptised in the church. In all this, you offered unwavering support.

However, as you built those dams, bridges, and ridges name it for him to become independent, something drastic happened. Your calabash fell, and the milk spilt. You were left with a broken gourd. All the empire you built around your son; you saw it crumbling.

You two as a couple lost your son in a terrible motor accident that not only robbed you as a father and mother but the siblings, wife, children lost the only gourd carrying the milk that had shade off its umbilical cord from the two of you.

I am sure you were left naked, you felt hopeless. His death created a ripple effect in the family, community and the entire country at its infancy when about to acquire independence. All these happened all of a sudden before any 'infant' becoming a-somebody.

You were robbed of a son you had educated to become a-somebody, to help you but now lay lifeless in front of you. What do you do? Is still my question. Having become naked as a result of this loss, you had your thinking caps on, and you never looked back as a terrible loss but as a chapter read and closed, beginning a new venture, a new unknown, that was really unknown.

You never gave up this hope of continuing to deliver your long-held hope and ambition of putting your family above everything else. You once again stood up and were counted. You became the anchor, the pivotal pole for everyone to hold on to. You made the impossible, possible, you made the unlikely, likely, you rallied a war cry and the soldiers matched along to your call.

You had well settled, planned retirement life and neat family organisation in Namwanga Village. You gave up all that, but you shouldn't have. Why did you?

I was reminded by my brother '*Mythical Bwenge*' that your sacrifice is equated to the Biblical story of '*mythical Abraham*' who was instructed by God to take a certain angle and decisions and ended up in the '*mythical wilderness*' but all ended '*mythically well*'. What a '*mythical coincidence*' in mirroring the two mythologies of you with Abraham's Biblical '*mythical journey*' in the book of Genesis.

In my appreciation, you had what it takes to make a decision. Your decision was that you uprooted yourselves from that ancestral land at Namwanga village and moved with your whole family to settle in Lwala P'Obona village where your son had acquired land that was barely two years old unto his death, where he had relocated his young family. You did not move in haste, but you moved without a wink.

In all thoughts, you would have opted to relocate this infant family and your son's lifeless body back to Namwanga the ancestral Land to be interred and family relocation back there too. You overlooked all this enormous authority you had and instead preferred to inter your son in his own newly acquired land. Oh my God, that was a great decision and sacrifice.

In the process, you decided to move away from the ancestral land into this new land of the unknown, where were you expected hostilities, but you stood your ground. You moved your entire homestead with all your children and great-grandchildren to camp and start a new life in this new place. You were like nomads as you left your permanent settled life with permanent structures and moved where you interred your son. Bless you, for that.

In death, I praise you for that as I would not envisage people would do such a thing and sacrifice a lot for the benefit of a few. May the good Lord grant you the Eternal Peace you two rightly deserve. I would never imagine someone making such a sacrifice, but you did.

This in return has taught me a very good lesson in my lifelong learning of making sacrifices to attain an intended or unintended goal, however difficult the situation may be dire, there is always light at the end of the tunnel. If you hit a brick-wall you know that is just the beginning of making sacrifices for the intended or unintended outcome. Perseverance is the key, so you taught me.

You two have taught me that great wisdom in what you did. I am just not sure whether your shoes could fit me but I will try as I too

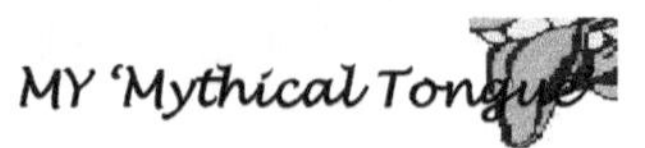

walk this similar treacherous journey, tracing laces of our sacrifices as I too lost the eldest son with a similar name and interred at the same place you rightly, safely and jealously guarded. I would have buried him in the United Kingdom. There was no need to have carried a lifeless corpse to be interred in Lwala P'Obona village. But on hindsight now, it was your ancestral *'mythical call'* that helped me carry out the similar ritual that you once did to have brought my son to the same place you interred your son. It came from one war cry that still echoes in my brain to-date when *'Mythical Nyari Ochido'* received my call about the death and all she asked me was, 'are you bringing the body for burial here'. I told her Yes. She then said that was all she wanted to hear and switched off the phone.

I cannot imagine leaving a corrugated Iron sheet house and moving into a grass-thatched house. Phew!!!!!!!!!!!! my heart up to you two. What a blessing I had. Do you think I would leave my London lifestyle and settle in Lwala P'Obona, time is the essences as I travel this similar journey, for I know you are there holding my hands.

If I may ask the two of you even in your Eternal Sleep, what were you thinking when you migrated with 24 children in total, herds of cattle and goats into this bewildering environment. What was your own thought process? If you cannot answer now, we shall be with you soon God bless. We shall compare notes and crack these jokes.

To be continued

JesseA

15

An Open Letter To My Mythical Sister-In-Law, My Other Mother, Jenny.

03/07/2019

Hey!! Mum Jenny

I know it was never easy coming into a family of the grownup children who loved cuddling around themselves, for that history gave them that destiny. You managed to walk into this *'mythical muddle puddle'* and fitted in so *'mythically well'*. You became part of the *'mythical team'*, part of the culture. You learnt all our strengths and weaknesses and worked around them so well. Where you felt you could panel beat the faults you did it with precision and never gave a toss. Where you felt you needed to strengthen the team you never shied away from giving your all positively. You became the pillar that was missing in my brother, the one formerly known as Seven Thirty.

You became his *'mythical anchor'* and in return, you supported him in trying to sustain the areas of his struggles in life. I know it was not easy, but who says coming into a home where everyone is either a brother or sister whatever the parentage is easy penetrating in. You were and still up to now continued pursuing the same actions you started with. I am so grateful that you supported me as a person to make me what I am today. I

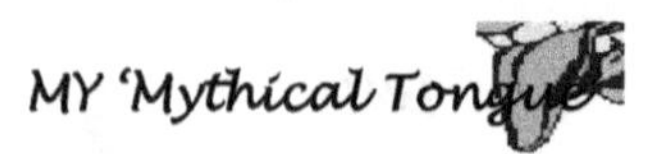

personally know I was not that easy, though it is hard for me to so admit.

I know I was your '*...Kichwa Mbaya...*' [bad head Swahili speak].

But you know what! Since my childhood, my head has always been the key and point of discussion at home. I don't know how you easily diagnosed that. I was also given that nickname '*...Thombo...*' [meaning hardened mud Japadhola speak]. As if that was not enough, they added '*...Nyarienga...*' [meaning pumpkin Dhopadhola speak] on top of '*...Thombo...*' Thus, it became '*...Thombo Nyarienga...*' Imagine carrying all those heavyweight names and then you add yours. Pew!! What a name.

When you were introduced into the home you entered this '*mythical quagmire*' of the '*mythical JopAlecho*' and '*mythical JopaSaulo*' and those two are no easy lot. I remember my maternal grandmother Phoebe [once said that in '*...iwoni itingo wich jowi...*' meaning you, yourself have carried the head of buffalo. You know how big the buffalo head is. In this regard, it meant that if you bring your own '*...wich jowi...*' [buffalo's head] you had to carry it.

Hence you got married into this '*mythical mire*' whereby you had to carry this '*...wich jowi...*' thing. I remember too your mum who is our mother in law warning you that you had carried this '*...wich jowi...*' but don't go back to '*mythical Kasubi Hill*' that mbu!! this thing has '*mythically defeated me*'. To-date, you have proved you are the '*mythical master*' of that '*mythical destination*' and you can '*mythically manoeuvre*' even the '*mythical hardest rock*'. You know what I could not '*mythically believe it*' that you could even soften and melt our '*mythical 'commander''* to the point of being good and submissive. That was and is an art I tell you '*mythically hysterical*'.

You were indeed the pioneer of creating this '*mythical conversation*' of sealing the '*...Banamawanga...*' [Luganda meaning outsiders] and the '...*Jumagara*...', [dhopadola mean a Muganda or with similar dialects] and or 'Juwiloka' [dhopadhola meaning outsiders]. Such was that marked deference's that were physically visible in these two families you ended up in. There would be talks of that one is a '...*Jamagara*...' or '...*Jawiloka*...' You brought that to an end. You also transcended the mythology of getting out of the comfort zone of '...*Jamagara*...' and becoming '...*Japecho*...' [meaning home owner].

To-date if you look at the whole concept and composition of the two families you came into; you have literary changed the perception and there are plenty of '...*Jumagara*...' littered all over the families and this is all due to you showing them and us that all is possible. I remember when you came in to settle you were given full responsibility for the whole family. You were told the parents were retiring and now it was your turn to take over. You did not shudder or look back to say I would not take this or that responsibility or should take the shortest cut because that loophole was already closed remember!! you remember!!!.

I remember when you tried to instill discipline and you sent one of my siblings to go to Kitoro Market at Entebbe Town and buy '...*Endagala*...' [banana leaves Luganda speak]. He turned around and said he does not understand Luganda and would not know how to say when he reached the market. However, you made him go anyway. He was defeated and came back with '...*endagala*...' Merely he was trying to avoid carrying this '...*endagala*...' along the way especially being seen by the other teenage sides of things.

I remember when you had just been thrown in the midst, we were told that from now on you were the sole person to be fully responsible to manage our affairs. I remember one time walking into the room and asking my brother for some money he turned

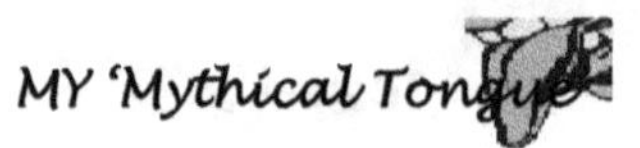

around and said he did not have anything, but I should ask you. I stood there for a few seconds dumbfounded, and I remembered what was told to us sometime back.

This also reminded me of how my parents brought us up to ask our mothers for anything, not them. To even my grandparents it was their nature to allow the women to take overall control of the homestead. Hence, I had to get used to it. I learnt and it made me learn more than learning. In fact, it made life look real. To-date, you are still the same self no changes. You are still on that path of steady progress keep it on impart to others too.

Thank you

To be continued

JesseA

16

An Open Letter To My Mythical Sister I Call My Swallah Sister

07/09/2018

Hey!! Swallah Sister

I hope this letter finds you well and '*mythically kicking*' as always in your newfound land. In fact, when I got out this pen to write to you this Open Letter tears flowed down my cheeks. I am aware you know why. It was not the tears of sorrows but of joy that at long last I could pen you this letter in the '*mythical true spirit*' of sister and brotherhood.

I always tell people that we can be '*mythical relatives*' but to turn a '*mythical relative*' into a friend needs crafting '*mythically*'. I am gladly stating that apart from being related we are indeed friends. It is, therefore, justifiable for me to pen this letter to you in the true spirit of friendship.

I have often wondered why we have anchored together this much. The explanation has not been fully coming my way. Hopefully, when you receive this letter you will write back and give me any background information that I may not have known to-date.

I have never ever written to you before, so this being my first written letter to you, I believe it is our shared history that I will not mention initially in this letter. However, as you open up, I will mention in the later letters as we communicate.

I am aware you have always protected me in this wildness of the unknown you have been there looking after me as my little sister. You have been and is an anchor of my other mother. Likewise, it seems subconsciously I look after you; I just do it out of my wits and whims. It is only when I have done it that is when I say oops!! And I ask myself, did I do that, and how did I do it. But I will have done it anyway.

As you know sometimes things happen but when you are asked for the reason why it happened there is often no answer to the question as there is often a blank sheet. It seems this has been our operation where answers lay in trails of blank sheets. It means it has happened and is the end of the story.

You know what? My Swallah!!. Today when I put this letter to you in writing, it touches the very soul of my reason to exist. It makes my heartthrob with the spirit of common bond that yearns for that touch of existence-hood.

I hope for a response if not received, and then I will still know that that window of contact is well and good open. See you soon.

To be continued

JesseA

17

An Open Letter To My Mythical Brother Formerly Known As Seven-Thirty.

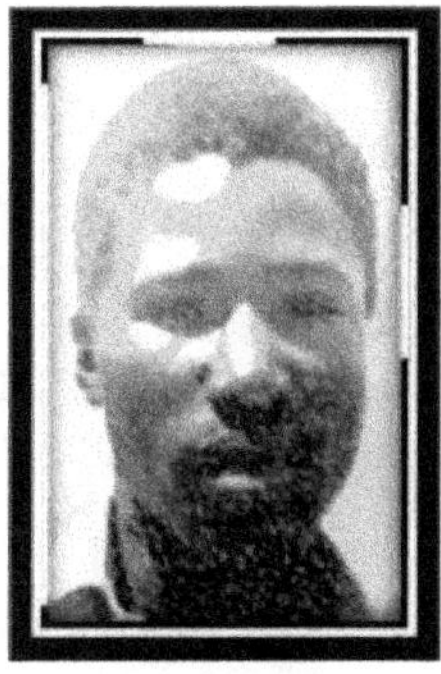

24/02/2019

Hey,!! Brother; Formerly known as Seven-Thirty.

What a journey that snakes around years on end. What a journey for all those decades of being at the forefront and driving seat of the family. You are such an asset; you are such oxygen, that everyone breathes by.

So, my brother formerly known as Seven-Thirty, welcome back. How was the journey in that flight-deck of the Boeing 787

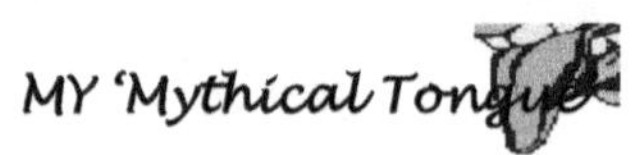

Dreamliner? I bet it was such an experience in that fantastic aircraft, which I understand has fuel efficiency and rides smoothly.

Reading about it and understanding from the horse's own mouth I get to know now that the aircraft is self-operated more so is it robotic and uses possibly the new technology of Artificial Intelligence. Was that the case? My understanding is that you went overtime for simulator checks and you were manoeuvring into how to fly that aircraft on taxiing, taking off, manoeuvres it while on-air and landing.

When I met you first prior to check-in for the *'mythical flight'* you beamed with smiles, no hesitations that you would fly that *'mythical aircraft'* having been air unworthy without airworthiness certificate for some time now.

When you took off and after a *'mythical successful flight'* you landed and when I met you at the *'mythical arrival lounge'* at the *'mythical airport'* you were, delighted and refreshed with an ear to ear smile.

Incidentally, if I may ask where that flight led you to, compared with Boeing 707. Anyway, maybe don't bother answering that as I know wherever you manoeuvre that aircraft to have been for all our good. Time immemorial is a test case.

Just a point of acknowledgement that you have been here long enough to nurture many into what they are today. You have toiled forever in pastures-Green, in *'mythical mountain-snowed'*, in the *'mythical desert sands'* but never gave a wink that you should stop. You have been through *'mythical tides'*, waves and still come out smiling.

You were born into a *'mythical culture'* of giving and not faltering. Some of us may never say thank you, as to say so would sort of wipe off the years of dedication and no compromise in giving and getting nothing in return. Indeed, you have given your whole. Who can doubt that possibly the insane?

May I ask you whether you have achieved that lifetime smile of achievements of a smiley face while giving, falling down, bruised, rising and still smiling and giving.

May I again ask the new *'mythical Sun-tan'* you got on that flight deck through those reflective windows, how does it feel to know there is a clear new bill of becoming a new you.

Having done *'mythical simulations'* and flown successfully that *'mythical Boeing 787 Dreamliner'*, having a nice time during your break for more successful flights wish you all the best. If you respond to my letter, I will be grateful. If you don't, I will continue poking you. Regards to all. I will be in touch.

To be continued

JesseA

18.

An Open Letter To My Mythical Brother Formerly Known As Seven-Thirty.

03/03/2019

Hey!!!,

They say a week in politics is a very long time. I know your busy schedule that is why you did not respond to my letter. However, as I earlier stated in my last post, I will keep poking you. I now know why you have not responded to my letter, but somehow someone was given a glimpse of how you have been busy hosting since you went on that inaugural flight in the Dreamliner. You might still be jetlagged. I understand some important people have been paying you visits.

Mbu!! I am told by none other than *'mythical Nyari Ochido Milyong'*[5] that *'mythical Grandma Tolofaina'* had made a flying visit sometime last week to see you, following your successful inaugural flight success. I understand that she was not happy that you did not tell her that you were being inducted into flying this new aircraft. I understand that somehow she came to know about it, so she had to make a swift journey via *'mythical Kenya Airways'* using the *'mythical Dreamliner 787'* into Heathrow and straight to your *'mythical place'*. You did not tell me, but I understand she came to pay you a courtesy call. According to this other sister of *'mythical Tolofaina'* who is also *'mythical Nyari Ochido Milyong'*,

[5] Grandma Tolofina's father [Nyari – infers the daughter of]

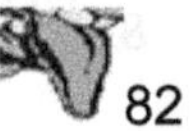

she said when *'mythical Tolofaina'* came back from her flying visit, she was very happy with your achievements. However, it seems *'mythical Tolofaina'* just sneaked out of the country to come and see you but never disclosed to anyone else about her coming.

When she went back, she popped by her sister's *'mythical Nyari Ochido'* late Thursday night into Friday morning and sneaked in her house to inform her of her successful trip. I guess she must have arrived in Nairobi City that early morning of Thursday and got into maybe a *'Chartered Mawingo'* bus or *'Akamba'* bus to arrive that late.

So, please, next time you are receiving such high-powered *'mythical delegation'* let some of us in the know. But anyway, what can we say, sometimes unannounced visits or unofficial visits are also part of the prerogative? So, I will not complain. I only hope you had a good chat and or may not share with us what you people discussed. I also hope you will now respond to my correspondences when you are less busy.

To be continued

JesseA

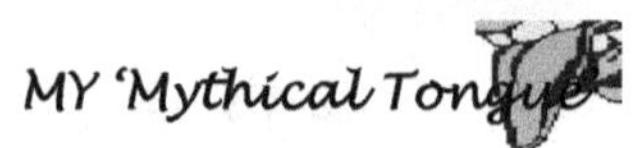

19

An Open Letter To My 'Mythical Brother 'The Flight Engineer.

07/08/2019

Hey!! Brother the Flight Engineer,

You remember those are one of your most cherished titles. It was one of your first professions. I hear you tried the *'mythical music trade'* but that it did not go according to plan. However, as you graduated into the adult life engineering skills took hold and you made it as one of the most successful flyers in your areas of expertise.

You initially graduated as an aeronautical engineer but eventually went into the flight mode. That is when you were chanced to have gone to the Queen's England. When you came back, we were all proud of you. But you know what you were such a *'mythical headache'* in a *'mythical good way'*. You were almost a delinquent child, a rebel with a cause for that matter. You were so mischievous in your own way. I am writing this up so that I can for once pull it out of the *'mythical closet'* for all the right reasons.

I remember your *'mythical Manjasi High School'* [MHS] days you were up to no good, you were such a rebel. No wonder you somehow carried it along to acquire another name the *'mythical 'Seven Thirty''*. Do you still remember when you were *'mythically expelled'* from Manjasi and it was damn God intervention that is how you were allowed back to school, and you finished it, oh!! my God. Otherwise, I don't know what would have happened to the flight engineer element of you, if that fate was not panel beaten in time. We thank God for that.

I remember one time I was chanced to escort you back to school and when we were in the '*mythical Tororo town*' you booked us into a bar called '*mythical Cozy Corner Bar*'. It was near '*mythical Hinnas Hotel*'. There was a jukebox blaring. So, you booked as there and; there were so many '*mythical female Tororo Girls School*' [TGS] around. The outstanding one was our dear sister Pusiika Aguga [RIP] (a daughter to Jafwonji Opoya Ragang - RIP) who became our family icon as a nurse in Entebbe Town whenever our health hours of need occurred. I saw this '*mythical jukebox*' thing someone throwing coins in it and pressing a '*mythical button*' then you could see how a row of '*mythical records*' running riot then one falls on the turntable and begins playing the chosen music. I tell you this was one of my wonders to this day how it was engineered.

That is how I knew what '*mythical beating life was*' I saw how a record was picked, thrown down that turntable and music blared. That was sweet, I am very grateful you showed me that. You see children never forget the little things you assume normal in life.

When you finished MHS, parents had wanted you to pursue Higher School Certificate [HSC] level like the Osinde Joma Pontius [RIP] who became our in-law. However, you had already gone to Nairobi city in Kenya to join the Apprentice training with the East African Airways [EAA]. You can imagine joining such a Corporation even before your Ordinary level Certificate results came out. You people used to brag about it as '*mythical CANTAB*'. Those were your '*mythical good old days*' you need to capture that with a glare.

Our parents called you back and had a prolonged discussion with you about coming back and joining the HSC level. You know what? You were so sneaky. You told parents it was okay you would be going back to Nairobi to pack up your bags and come back to pursue the Higher education. Anyway, the rest is history for instead you went up the sky and it became the limit.

Somehow, they say God works in mysterious ways. You pursued the courses and training with EAA in Engineering and at the dawn of you graduating and just about to enjoy your sweat of real employment, Uganda government was overthrown. Within a short time, the monies that were kept for us to pursue education and support were stopped by the military regime. The monies were deposited with the Administrator General, in the President's Office, whom Wanume Kibedi[6] was the one in charge.

We were all handed and herded over to you for financial assistance like upkeep, fees, feeding, clothing name them became your other *'mythical expenditures'*. You became a fully blown *'mythical father'* of I don't know how many *'mythical kids'* of all ages. You became an inspiration for I don't know how you managed it all without favours.

You turned a father figure overnight. Being in Nairobi City Kenya allowed us to go places though I remember my first trip when I had finished my Primary Leaving Exams [PLE]and had passed and admitted at Kiira College Butiki, you invited me and our brother Jero to come around. We used Akamba bus, on an overnight journey and arrived in Nairobi City into the morning. You were waiting for us and whisked us to your accommodation at Kileleshwa. You showed us what true Nairobi City *'mythical life'* was. It was the first time I went for a Movie or I call it to the Cinemas. We watched the movie where Charles Bronson was acting in. This made me begin to brag around when people asked me who my best actor was. Even in the autographs, it was my dream actors when mentioning it in mine or others autographs the present-day something called Facebook or Instagram.

You took us to one of the best hotels in Nairobi to have dinner. I ordered some food that turned out to have too much chilly. The

---

[6] Foreign Minister in Gen Idi Amin-Dada's regime 1971

first intake I sweated. My mouth was so hot that I'd to dash off at breakneck speed for a glass of ice-cold water but pretended to be enjoying the meal, regardless.

As part of my requirements to go back to school you bought me virtually all including a suit. I had one of the best metallic suitcases that was the envy of the school. You put me at a different level as in Uganda things were biting due to the regime change and economic war, or rather it was a *'mythical oil war'*.

You took us places including going into Embakasi Airport [present day Jomo Kenyatta Airport[7]] where you were flying in and out. You showed us where maybe a day before I wouldn't have dreamt of being in.

You remember while I was at Butiki I sort of became that bit of you while in your Manjasi days. I was about to be expelled from school. You sent to our parents your car a sleek Alfa Romeo for them to come and visit me and have contact with my headmaster the dreaded *'mythical Mr Musanyana'* [RIP] for he was also a friend to the late **I**srael **O**chwo **A**lecho [IOA] because they were both teachers who qualified from Kabwangasi Teacher Training College. I can now tell you that a can of worms was opened when they met us *'Musanyana'* almost wanted me to pack my bags and go back with them. He was so pissed off with me as he now knew who I was from the type of family he knew. Your Alfa Romeo saved the day and very grateful for that.

The second time I came back to Nairobi City just as we started enjoying again the ambience of Nairobi when all hell broke loose. An announcement was made that the East African Community[8] had ceased to exist; it had collapsed. Thanks to this, the EAA ceased trading. That was as devastating as the breadbasket, holes had been punched into and *'mythically drained'*. It was a trying moment. We left you with this *'mythical dilemma'* of where you

---

[7] Renamed after the post-independence first President of Kenya.

[8] An economic community of three countries - Uganda, Kenya and Tanzania

could go next, but looking now at your eyes then I would wonder how you felt when you had all these burdens to carry them through with signs of unemployment at *'mythical short notice'*.

Being you, brushed off the disappointments, packed your bags and came back to Uganda. By then the Uganda Airlines had been started by Amin Dada[9] and this is partly what led to the collapse of EAC and EAA, though there is a bigger picture too to it, so I hear.

You came back and found our late Uncle, my *'mythical uncle Captain David Omitta'* [RIP][10] of the Uganda Airforce who persuaded you to come back and serve Uganda Airlines, and you camped at his place as you settled in. You then started working for Uganda Airlines[11]. You remember those trip journeys you people were making with Boeing 707 full of coffee and by-passing the embargo imposed on the regime. You could see the Boeing 707 taking off with a bellyful of coffee being taken to Djibouti and in return bringing back to the regime the essentials required for the regime sustainment. Eventually, Entebbe Town became our second home again as you settled and was fully employed by Uganda Airlines.

I wanted to ask you that being in the airlines you were *'mythically flying places'* and eating all types of foods what made you not like eating grass? as you called it! Meaning salads defeats me. That one I leave you to offer me an answer if we happen to meet.

However, our times in Entebbe were memorable. You brought to us our sister-in-law who became another mother in the home. Thanks for that for the choice well executed. You started offering all the unwavering support to all of us and did it with extraordinary zeal and selfless generosity.

---

9 President of Uganda 1971-1979 – military rule.

10 Airforce Mig-21 Jet Pilot 1977-1989

11 Started 1977 - post East African Airways/East African Community.

But remember you became a *'mythical somebody'* else too, around this time. You were a *'mythical silent burner'*. You acquired a new hidden name being called *'mythical Seven-Thirty'*.

When I came to know what was behind the name Seven-Thirty, it made me laugh. A whole airline Flight Engineer who likes keeping time to be bang on time on flights yet when certain things were needed from him, he could state, I will be there by seven-thirty but ends up using the "African Time".

Anyway, it worked somehow, and you managed to create those structures that necessitated the regime change and so I hear you became a Ugandan President for a day. So, what happened after that? Was it an overthrow? I think I am waiting for that book to be written in: - *'A day as a President for one day Only'*.

You supported us and another issue became of you and family. You had to leg it at short notice leaving behind all you had worked for all you had tried to build in Uganda and all you needed to be. You were not going to look for *'mythical pastures'* anew but protect your blood being spilt. Somehow you managed to make it and I know that being who you are it was a difficult time for you, but you never lounged still. You dusted yourself off and started a new. If I could write a book about you just with the word 'determination' I would fill *'mythical Tolofaina's granary'*.

You tried to get back into the airline industry until you felt it was time to hang up those gloves. You moved into the social science field and continued to survive and support the family within and without far and wide. You continued being the *'mythical eye'* of all of us, then we lost our brother *'mythical Jero'* under your stewardship in London. I know it was not easy, but you rallied the troops.

The few things you have implanted in me are one of always looking at things from the positives. You do not allow the negatives to pin you down and define who you are. The last one I hold dear to date is the one that you sat me down and *'mythically told me'* straight

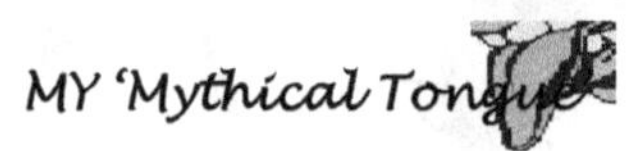

into my *'mythical eyes'* at that time when I was so low when darkens happened at noon, in that flat at that address you walked with me and said that "*...Jesse, do not go into competition with anybody...*"

Since then anything I do, I reflect on it as before I say a word, utter a word or do anything? I ask is what I am doing, going to say would it conflict with what you warned me on "*do not go into competition with anybody*". This is where the *'mythical tongue'* resurrected to begin playing a very significant role in me. You are such an ancestral *'mythical geek'*!!

I, therefore, need to report back that since then I have reduced my levels of known stresses of life you can rightly avoid. It has made me get into the grip of understanding that word *'competition'*

I am happy to let you know that since then, I have now added something on top of that. I have stopped even competing with my *'mythical self'* as it will be self-defeating because it is still a competition in myself, my inner thoughts my own doing etc.

Keep on doing things the way you view to the *'mythical eyes'* of your *'mythical ancestors'* as I believe they are your *'mythical inspirations'* and please thank them to have offered you the *'mythical tools'* to do things differently to better the levels they were at. I hope you get the right *'mythical Stool'* that is hidden in the *'Mythical Afrika Habitat'*!! *'Mythical Jackson speaks'*. I thank you for *'mythically walking'* with me in the last two years and it will carry me through. I know your door is always *'mythically open'* do not shut it to me or anybody else. You *'mythically mean well'*.

To be continued

JesseA

20

An Open Letter To My 'Mythical Sister' Who Is Silently Called "Commander"

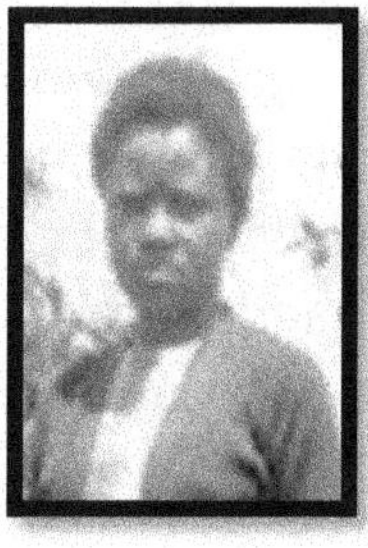

05/03/2019

Hey! Oops? Commander,

It was never meant to never ever come to the public fora. It was always a silent whisper, sort of sworn in secrecy like the *'mythical Freemasonry*[12]*'*. All of us have been calling you Commander since time immemorial. I know as you always say, "I am shocked" and so you should be shocked now you know you are called the commander. I could not contain this *'mythically sworn secret'* by

[12] https://en.wikipedia.org/wiki/Freemasonry

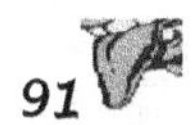

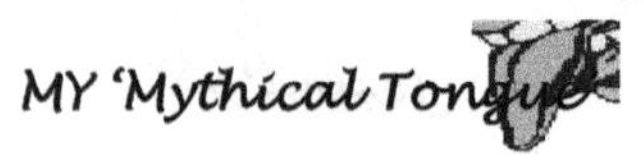

anyone who has had contact with you and stayed within your realm of authority.

I know all my *'mythical siblings'* and the like know I will get a bollocking from them as I have now let the *'mythical cat'* out of the *'mythical bag'* and they know now; I am going to *'mythically pay'* for it because they can no longer hide around the name when discussing you.

You know what I had to openly come out and tell you to your own face so that you should know it as others seem to be taking the mantelpiece from you and I need to run fast to expose our era who was our commander in chief of our civilian forces. You know what as others are coming in, they will begin asking us to show them our *'mythical generals'* and if we don't expose our 'Commander' today they will begin with those words your granddaughter told you the other day.

You remember when we had a *'mythical chat'* and you stated that you are now being called 'fake' really *'mythically fake'*. I could not sleep my nights through well as I kept thinking: "How dare they call our *'mythical General Commander'* 'Fake'?"

Indeed, you *'mythically accepted'* that with a *'mythical laugh'* not knowing you have been *'mythically commanding civilian forces'* for close to sixty *'mythical years'*. It seems your commanding tactics is waning no wonder your granddaughter sees you as *mythical* fake.

I wonder how this *'mythical granddaughter'* saw this new *'mythical you'*. Anyway, I leave that story for another day. However, before I move on, I am still seething, and I would advise you to go back to your *'mythical granddaughter'* and tell her you are not fake.

You have commanded your forces during the periods when a 'Slate' was used for writing on using White Chalk, unlike now when they use an iPad[13].

You were *'mythically commanding your forces'* in an era when *'mythical 'Quink Ink''* and *'mythical 'Parker pens''* were used for writing unlike now when ballpoint pens and the computer have taken over.

You commanded forces in the era of the *'mythical gramophone, radiogram, telex, fax, record players'* name it. Tell them they would never know what an autograph is.

Tell her you to have a lot to handover all tangible and original, not their current world where it is *'mythically indistinguishable'* of what is *'mythical fake'* and not fake.

On another note, I just realised that you have been *'mythically overthrown'* as "*Mythical Commander-in-Chief*". Until I attended a handover ceremony that occurred in London on 28th of August 2018, when it was disclosed by none other than your dad that you were the *'mythical 'Och''* who declared that *'mythical 'Miss-N''* had been all along also being silently called *'mythical Commander'* what a coincidence. It was disclosed that she was also called in silence as *'Mythical Commander-in-Chief'* for donkey years in hiding and up to now, no one dared say it in front of her. It, therefore, beggars' belief how commanders are actually feared, and people cannot dare call them so. Yet a Commander commands battalions and they should know what their roles are.

Anyway, in military terms, once tipped as a *'mythical commander'* you cannot be stripped of the rank, even in retirement. So, tell your *'mythical granddaughter'* you are not *'mythically fake'* because you are still a *bonafide 'mythical Commander-in-Chief'* even if they are forcing you into this so-called *'mythical retirement'*. Even your *'mythical 'Miss-N''* is now the new exposed Commander-in-Chief. What the Jupadhola say *"Tucho winyo dhu'mach"* meaning mentioning the bird near the fire, you could easily lose the bird before that fire.

---

13 https://en.wikipedia.org/wiki/IPad

In this context, raising expectations about what is to be eaten before knowing that the food to be eaten is there. I hope I will not face the firing squad. I am only a messenger. So, do not shoot me; I am just conveying it the way it is.

To your granddaughter: Tell her you are not a fake commander but a real one who has commanded battalions in all wars for close to sixty years being retired but and still effective does not make you fake.

In your old commanding days, you were a no-nonsense Commander. You would have told your granddaughter the way you one time told your sister Tina (Min'Awino) when she failed to obey you that you would climb with her over our Lwala P'Obona homestead into the other side. And you know what happened? She cowed. Such were your tactical manoeuvres. So, my silent commanding sister what is happening now that you seem to readily accept the little fake. Toughen up, get your *'mythical boots'* on, put on your *'mythical fighting gear'* and continue doing your *'mythical work'* as *'mythical Commander-in-Chief'*. Lastly, stiffen your *'mythical back'*.

I hope you will get back to me soon.

Regards to all

To be continued

JesseA

21

An Open Letter To My 'Mythical ABBA Sister 'My Tina Awino

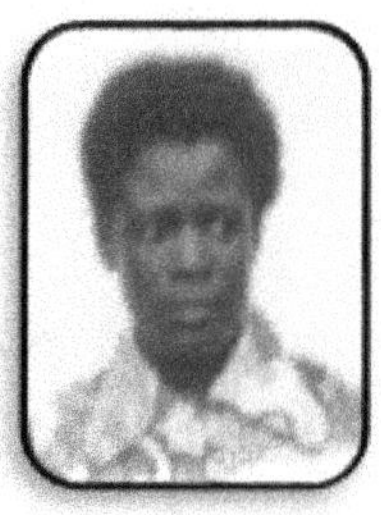

22.06.2019

Hey!! Tina,

You have continued being on my *'mythical mind'* though long gone. You sing in my *'mythical brain'* like all the *'mythical ABBA songs'*[14]. You are like a 'Chiquitita'[15] to me. You are like the *'mythical song'* and its *'mythical lyrics'*. I will always remember you by:

> *Chiquitita, tell me what's wrong*
> *You're enchained by your own sorrow*
> *In your eyes there is no hope for tomorrow*

---

14 https://en.wikipedia.org/wiki/ABBA.

15 https://www.google.com/search?q=lyrics+of+chiquitita&sourceid=ie7&rls=com.microsoft:en-US&ie=utf8&oe=utf8 accessed15/04/2020

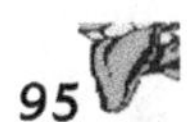

How I hate to see you like this
There is no way you can deny it
I can see that you're oh so sad, so quiet
Chiquitita, tell me the truth
I'm a shoulder you can cry on
Your best friend, I'm the one you must rely on
You were always sure of yourself
Now I see you've broken a feather
I hope we can patch it up together
Chiquitita, you and I know
How the heartaches come and they go and the scars they're leaving
You'll be dancing once again and the pain will end
You will have no time for grieving
Chiquitita, you and I cry
But the sun is still in the sky and shining above you
Let me hear you sing once more like you did before
Sing a new song, Chiquitita
Try...

Whenever this *'mythical ABBA'* new song came out you made us listen to it, wind, unwind, rewind the tape until you had written down all the lyrics of the song. Sometimes the *'mythical tape'* could twist. You made sure we got it out of the tape did a *'mythical pen spin and unspin'*. Did *'mythical finger tweaking'* to bring the tape back to *'mythical life'*. You were such an enigma to us whenever you walked into a room it became *'mythically vibrant'*. It became *'mythically radiant'*. Your *'mythical warmth'* could fill the room with fresh air *'mythically as you were the smile of the family'*.

You never minded doing the jobs that *'mythical donkeys'* do. No wonder you kept the *'mythical faith'*. When you were employed at the Standard Chartered Bank, which was in the middle of Kampala city. It was the easiest place to reach. You were in such a strategic place for easy reach. It meant everyone or anything could reach you. The reaching was more to do with simple requirements for transport, cigar, food, fees, name them. You could just smile, walk away and come back with something. It was as if you owned the bank. No one knew that behind that persona, that smile, that generosity you could have just gone away to borrow to give to the John and Mary.

You were indeed like your namesake who could give to the hungry even in times of adversity. I remember one time while sharing your good memories, my brother-in-law said whenever he came back from the UK after his enjoyment etc., he could just walk to you and ask you for just that fare to drop him off at Entebbe International Airport to catch his flight and you didn't wink but just went behind came back offered the needful and all was well.

You remember when we were young in that early childhood at Lwala P'Obona village. Trekking on every morning going to that Siwa primary school, looking for the elusive education. Do you remember when you could wake us up to give us breakfast, wash our legs? Push us ahead of you to go to school on time and not be late. You were that inspiration. You were that icon.

You were the sister who tried to dry everyone's moisty eye. You were the sister who offered shelter at the point of need. Sometimes I sit down and think you were the sister who became the donkey offering shelter when it rained heavily. You were the sister who was prepared to stand on the verandah to offer the wandering humanities space. You were the sister who could stand in for others; who could die on other's behalf.

I will remember to this day you are the *'mythical sister'* who saved my *'mythical life'* on that day at that time when it *'mythically mattered most'*. That was the second time as I remember my *'mythical life'* was saved. The first one as you remember was done by that *'mythical AMO's Government'* offering us that *'mythical 'Omwana Akaba''*. On this occasion, you indeed made the final decision and didn't ask me for my *'mythical thoughts'* but told me to get into the car and come along with you. How it all went I don't know but you made the impossible look like just a speck.

The last words I heard from you while on your last days on this earth were uttered when I rang you. You told me that Jesse *'kech nekani'*. Meaning Jesse, I am hungry. That one caused my heart to miss some beats. It was so devastating that it made me cry. To this day I hold that dear till we meet again.

To be continued

JesseA

22

An Open Letter To My Mythical Brother Jero.

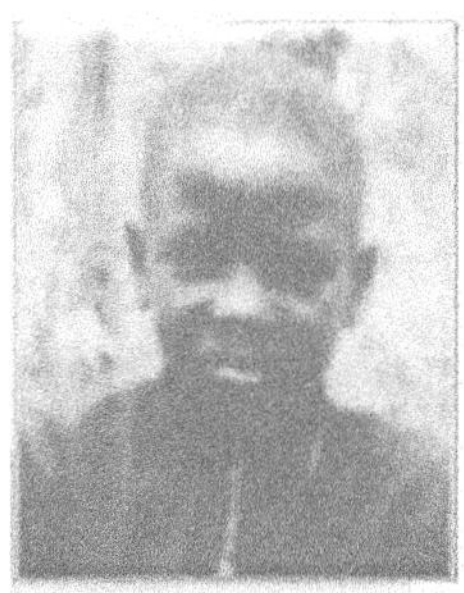

28/11/2017

Dear Mythical Brother Jero,

Where can I begin? Should I begin as my '*mythical childhood best friend*'? Should I begin as my '*mythical best sibling*'? Should I begin as my '*mythical adult best friend*'? Should I begin as my best mentor? I cannot settle for less. You were '*mythically everything*' to me.

You were my shield, You were my anchor;

You were the inner soul that left and left me empty inside and hollow.

With all this hollowness and emptiness where can I begin, when I have been swept under my feet my this '*mythically unknown phenomenon*'. Well under this '*mythically unknown*' let me

 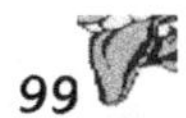

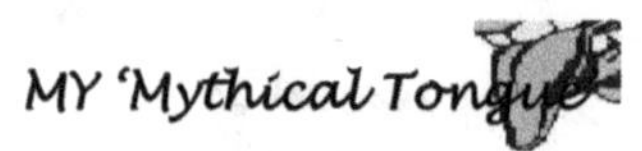

capture from somewhere where memory lane flows like the *'mythical River Nile'* snaking from the heartbeat of our *'mythical Africa'* through the arteries of *'mythical Africa'* and pouring all the *'mythical African'* soils into the *'mythical Mediterranean plain' which became the 'mythical Mediterranean Sea'*.

The preceding and follow-up captures the concept of the *'mythical Noah'* building his *'mythical Ark'* to save that *'mythical Afrika Flora and faunae'*[16].

All the *'mythical attractive outcomes'* helping the *'mythical European species'* paving the *'mythical streets'* with *'mythical Gold'* and the trees flowering *'Mythical Gold'* ready for *'mythical picking'*. The *'mythical streets'* and *'mythical Golden Trees'* built and fertilised using *'mythically silted top-soils'*, carried away from our *'mythical beautiful country'*, Uganda, through the arteries of Africa.

My *'mythical brother Jero'* ensured I was silted through to meet him in this upper thrust of this *'mythical universe'*. Such was the love of my brother. I realised the once *'mythical history'* of *'Mythical Africa'*[17] learning about *'Mythical Europe'* and *'Mythical Europe'*[18] learning about *'Mythical Africa'* was *'mythically faulty'* as there was this *'mythical belief'* that *'mythical Europe'* discovered the *'mythical River Nile'* and yet I was fully *'mythically there'* all along, imagine!.

My *'Mythical brother Jero'*, do you still remember the 07/11/1990 when, 'I', one of the *'mythical Ugandan Nile Silt'* landed at the *'mythical Heathrow'*? What a reference point to start from! That was a journey by the *'mythical Ugandan Crane'* that trekked like the *'mythical Nile river'* pouring its *'mythical silt'* into the *'mythical Thames waters'*, what a *'mythical irony'*.

---

16 https://en.wikipedia.org/wiki/Noah's_Ark
17 Africa Learns About Europe – H.W.R Hawes. Pub: Longmans, Arusha 1960.
18 Europe Learns About Africa – Book 1. J.B.Whithead. Pub: Longmans 1960

You are such a star that shone and continue to shine in people's minds. You remember how you came and whisked me away like a *'mythical VIP'*, jumping on the passenger side in a *'mythical car registration PEG 5 X a Camry'*? Whatever that meant to me at the time created a-thinking what your *'mythical car'* registration PEG was.

Your *'mythical whirlwind drive'* snaked me into a *'mythical motorway'* that perplexed my *'mythical mind'* twisted my *'mythical soul'* embraced my *'mythically new-found freedom'* echoing my *'mythical mother's'* words of the *'mythical pen and paper'*.

Do you still remember that car, your *'mythical Camry'*, that snaked its way into the *'mythical London streets'* carrying your *'mythical VIP'* who came from a *'mythical Shithole Country*[19] where there was no *'mythical cars bumper'* to bumper?

You snaked your *'mythical PEG 5 X'* car through the streets with *'mythical traffic lights'* turning like as if I was in a *'mythical Ugandan hall disco'* with turning *'mythical blinkering lights'* of all shades. That was *'mythically amazing'*, really fascinating, especially coming from a *'mythical country'* where *'mythical police'* stand in the middle of the road to give drivers directions.

You then landed me in a town called Brixton. Oh! My *'mythical brother'*, you were such a good coach. You told me just enter that *'mythical building'* and say this and that and like as if a *'mythical hole in the wall'*; a *'mythical Queens'* head appeared.

We again entered PEG 5 X and you drove me off into a *'mythical wonderful mansion'*. *'Mythical Keys'* clicked and clacked. This was 104 Brixton Hill. If you can imagine the *'mythical Muyenga Hill'*, Mbuya Hill, Kololo Hill; This was a *'mythical world-class Hill'*; Brixton Hill and a *'mythical Mansion' to crown it all.*

---

19 https://www.theguardian.com/us-news/2018/dec/26/from-shithole-countries-to-a-private-agreement-trumps-2018-lowlights

 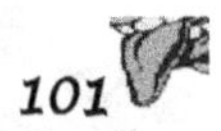

I could not believe that it was just that '*mythical yesterday*' I was '*mythically airborne*' from my Shithole country snaking in the sky via another '*mythical shithole country*' that has an airport called '*mythical Embakasi*'.

I remember in the 1970's we used only to go and see the '*mythical entrance*' of this airport when either picking or dropping off another '*mythical brother*' who kept off carrying some rectangular '*mythical black leather case*'. I do not know whether to call it a briefcase because it was not '*mythical brief-suitcase*' but there were no suits in them. Okay, let me settle for a case because at least it carried voluminous books that; I didn't make head or tail. As for me, I was used to having a student case carrying all sorts of network materials to and from school. He was a '*mythical Flight Engineer*' whatever that meant at the time. I was proud that day that I was at the other end of '*mythical Embakasi Airport*' jumping or hopping from one '*mythical plane*' to another, like my '*mythical brother*' the '*mythical Flight Engineer*'. Only that I had a '*mythical Black handy bag*' carrying basics. Anyway, that will be another '*mythical story*' for another day, let us stick to the script.

When my '*mythical brother*' Jero opened the Mansion, I was wowed gapping like a '*mythical Ape*', if I was in a Shithole Country, the '*mythical flies*' would take immediate '*mythical refuge*' in my '*mythical mouth*'.

Straight away my '*mythical brother*' took me to have a '*mythical jacuzzi bath*'! He took me through a flight of stairs into what was called a Penthouse.

To my surprise, I had this introduction. He introduced me, "Jesse, this is my '*mythical landlord*'. He owns the whole of this '*mythical property*' and has other property portfolios".

My Brother's Landlord welcomed me and made me feel welcome and at home in a moo!!. He made me feel very comfy and assured me that my stay will be fine and he blessed me. This became one of my memorable days and moments in a new country and new culture.

My brother's landlord became my *'mythical landlord'*; and made a great impact on my *'mythical life'*. He signed me into the *'mythical penthouse'* and would eventually offer me several *'mythical accommodations'* in and around London until he finally settled me into the current accommodation of my liking. This is how this best *'mythical Muganda landlord'*, I came to know in my life. He *'mythically intertwined'* himself into the fabric of my life like threadworms, only that I did not get diarrhoea or dysentery. My *'mythical Muganda landlord'* was a dominant figure in my brother's life. That I will give you an insight later. For now, let me continue to give you a glimpse of my *'mythical Brother Jero'*. He played his role in modelling me into life in a new culture.

You know what memories flash and spirits leave on. You *'mythically breathed'* your last *'mythical free oxygen'* in April 1995 at that *'mythical hospital St Thomas Hospital London'* where *'mythical Nurse Florence Nightingale'* practised her nursing You lived short of your birthday that fell on the 18/04/1995. I will cherish every moment as you left me with a wonderful landlord who became my *'mythical Landlord'* and my best friend too.

To be continued
JesseA

23.

An Open Letter To My Mythical Landlord Leo /

29/11/2017

Dear My Mythical Landlord Leo.

Whatever happened to our first love when you showed me the property that you had newly built. You made me feel comfy. I hosted the best house-warming party that people are still talking about. I will cherish it until that day.

You made me like your attitude towards building to rent for the needy and dispossessed. You made me feel that you were there for me and likes of me. You made me sign along the dotted line a long-term lease agreement that tied me to you and bonded me to your vision of helping the future.

Your love for me soothed my burning heart as I felt the desire to support you in your project of landlord acquisition and becoming a renowned architect of property acquisition and property mogul as such.

From time to time you came and we reviewed the tenancy and you could move round to see what was wrong and what was right.

You would often put everything right. "Right Now," as was your middle name.

To put everything right, to address all my concerns right from nothing to everything. You often surprised me by forfeiting even '*mythical three months*' rent-free whenever you felt like it. You often gave me that little breathing space to have my issues addressed and you wouldn't call those rent arrears but rent-free. Such was your friendship with your tenant.

You alleviated my mirror of dispossession. You more-or-less looked and sounded like the African Uganda's British Richard Branson of my Virgin Housing.

I anticipated that my long-term relationship with you would be cemented in this accommodation. I began by acknowledging that your income stream through the rental you offered me would shine on our long-term commitment and relationship.

Time passed and I paid my dues. Time passed and you started ignoring your responsibilities. However, I continued with my obligations. The once wonderful house turned into a nightmare. Disrepair became the norm.

"Disrepair" now replaces *"Right Now"* as your middle name.

The central heating system became historical as if it was the Victorian era. It reminded me of sleeping at an African funeral in the wet season and the only place to seek shelter when it is cold, or rain is a hut that fits only 3 people including pots pans and a pot of drinking water including chicken, goats and of course all those things you can imagine.

The boiler saw its day yesterday like a '*mythical African burnt ash*', waiting for it to be shoved into a makeshift pot to make '*mythical Soda ash*'.

The once-glittering tiled rooftop that shone in Summer welcoming the sun moving from the tropics to the northern hemisphere faded further north in the Antarctic's. The once tiles that blessed the '*mythical winter weather*' and the piles of snow became an eyesore in the neighbourhood that even the local authority condemned it.

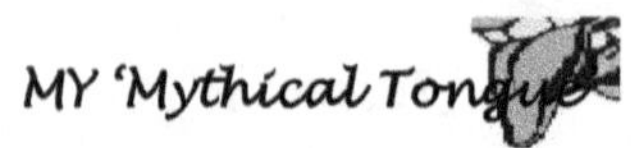

The once internal decor has seen the day with everything that glows have faded into the yesteryears, waiting for the crawlies to move in and make a home.

I remember a copied phrase that a *'mythical Good Muganda'* is a dead one. I realised that you being my *'mythical Landlord'*, come from the-*'mythical Buganda'* and as such fitted the Muganda mythology. To my understanding, it was coined and presented that it was a former *'mythical President of Uganda'* the late Dr Apollo Milton Obote[20], who said it. I have always dispelled this *'myth'*. The man himself married a *'mythical Muganda'* wife, who to-date has not died. Really, *'mythically speaking'* is she really a *'mythical Muganda'* a *'Mythical Kalule'*. The *'mythical Muganda'* wife became the mother of a *'mythical nation'* who supported her husband to hold the instruments of power in 1962 for Uganda to be an independent nation. Who can say that was not a *'mythical Good Muganda'* and she is not dead?

In my family by marriage or marrying, plenty of Baganda have littered the homestead and beyond like White Ants looking for the moon in the period when of harvest or Grasshoppers [Nsenene] spreading their wings. This has happened both in my tribe the *'mythical Jopadhola'* and us also infiltrating the *'mythical Buganda'* sphere[21].

As far as I am aware, they are all good *'mythical Baganda'* and neither side is dead. I hope I am *'mythically right'*. This is the very reason I trusted you like a *'mythical Muganda'* Landlord living in the United Kingdom who has been a prosperous property owner and a mogul as such.

I personally know you are one of the best Muganda I have ever met, but why have you done this to me? Not being in a position to

[20] Prime Minister of Uganda 1962-1965; President 1965-1971, and 1980-1985.
[21] https://en.wikipedia.org/wiki/Buganda

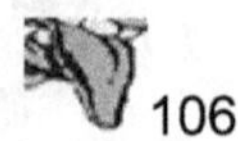

sort my dwelling the way you used to do. My life and that of my family is being threatened by your ineptitude.

We often agreed who should do what by when and how. I have on several occasions called you on phone but either it's switched off, not available or whenever you see my call you swipe the do not disturb button. I tried you on WhatsApp[22], but it seems you have blocked me because the two ticks do not show; it only shows one tick. We were once *'mythical Facebook[23] friends'*, but you blocked me there too. Whenever I do a search your name does not exist.

Because of *'mythical hypothermia'*, coupled with condensation, moulds growing on walls and windows as if it has become a house where we harvest moulds for the United Kingdom and Northern Ireland and European export. If you could support us to look for the market, then we would be filthy rich and be able to renovate your property. That is if there has been your primary purpose and intended outcome

Whenever I visit my doctors/GP my medical records are no longer Curriculum Vitae [CV] like it used to be. It now reflects as if it is a PhD fellow doing a thesis and a long list of citations based on the books, journals read, presented papers made at various seminars, universities.

To be continued

JesseA

22 https://en.wikipedia.org/wiki/Facebook

23 Ibid 19

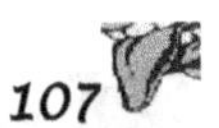

24

An Open Letter Response To My Mythical Landlord Leo.

01/12/2017

Dear My Mythical Landlord Leo

What a surprise when I sent that Open Letter to you. I thought you would ignore it and bury your head under the thick sand.

I woke up this morning and found that at last, you had *'mythically unblocked'* me on the WhatsApp. I saw all the messages that I sent you from eternity were all having double ticks. To my surprise, the double ticks were all to my surprise blue. Oh my!! Oops!! What a blessing for such a landlord to come out of his bunker, out of his limbo to come back and address my concerns. You brought me back to life as if I was reading Barack Obama's book *"Audacity of Hope"*[24].

You made my heart dance the '*mythical 'sixties twist''* not the 'seventies bumping' and I thought I was about to pass out. But, alas, it was an excitement of knowing the existence of my landlord. At last, I knew that I still had the best Muganda landlord. When your silent whisper came out with that phrase *"stick to him like*

[24] https://www.amazon.co.uk/Audacity-Hope-Thoughts-Reclaiming-American/dp/1847670830. https://en.wikipedia.org/wiki/Barack_Obama

Glue" did you mean superglue or this glue kindergarten children use of pasting paper.

Anyway, don't worry to answer my question. Glue is glue, is glue, it connects two or more things together and that is what matters *'mythically speaking'*. I am now connected to you like glue full stop. My heart is melting like a *'mythical melting pot'* of *'mythical honey'*. My *'mythical self-worth* has arisen as if it was is a *'mythical slain state'*. My *'mythical self-esteem'* has been *'mythically aroused'* as if I was in my *'mythical early years'* of having *'mythical teenage experiences'*.

Today I walked out of my house with a *'mythical swag'* knowing very well that I have at last have reclaimed you as the *'mythical landlord'* I have ever known. This is now forever. You will never again do a *'mythical disappearing act'*; the past is now behind us. The future holds us, dear. I will hold on to you as my last straw of hope like Obama's *'Audacity of Hope'*[25] book. I will hope on you as if there is no more *'mythical hope'* tomorrow.

I will pave for you the runway to my house so if you currently flying even 'Airforce One' it will be able to accommodate your needs but not wants.

I will then upon your landing tell you all about it for I know you might be holding on to some portfolio in the *'mythical Bank of England'*. You might be sitting on goldmine next to the *'mythical Bank Governor'* Mark Carney, so I think.

I am aware of your influence goes beyond *'mythical property development'*.

---

[25] Ibid 21

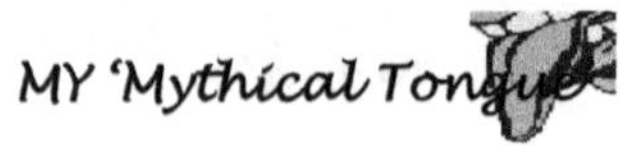

I am now begging for forgives I now know you still have the 'Right Now' attitude. I did not' know the power of Open letter can deliver immediate action as I can now see people beginning to put scaffolding around my house.

I respect you. OH! Did I say respect or fear? No, I said respect.

I don't fear you because you are a down to earth fellow.

I do respect you because you walk, breath, eat, sit and sleep with that aura of respect. I wonder how you cultivate such a thing called the aura.

To be honest, the only other person who has that cultivated aura was your '*mythical Brother-in-Law*', the Baganda call it MUKO, - The Late Milton Obote[26].

I know if I say more in this letter would be delaying workers doing the needful outside.

To be continued

JesseA

---

[26] Ibid 17

25

An Open Letter To Thank My Mythical Landlord Leo

02/01/2018

Dear My Mythical Landlord Leo

You are such a good-natured person. I remember when I first landed in the UK and how you did a lot to me. You remember you first introduced me to a job in the UK you were the all-rounder person.

Remember the Euro-Car Parts and how the Asian was good to you and me. Those were our fellow countrymen, Uganda-Asians. They were brought up from a humble background of Jinja industrial town. They were expelled by the then Uganda government under Idi Amin Dada. You educated me how they started from a car garage and then introduced spare parts and now purely selling car spares. They had a garage repair shop and went into selling spares and began a big warehouse that involved in the countrywide business.

We had our quality times there, as you know it. We were the cream of the other side, you know it. The Euro-Car Parts outgrew them and sold it off. But you know what you showed me how to mint pounds and how to save. You were so close that you nurtured me into the business of work-life. I knew from then that I had to hold on to your type of work ethics. It delivered results that, to-date, has littered my life on end. I thank you for that bleep of that choice you made to do that to me.

To be continued

JesseA

26

An Open Letter To My 'Mythical Friend' GOOK At KCB.

08/02/2018

Dear Mythical Friend GOOK from KCB,

I studied for my Ordinary Level secondary school at Kiira College Butiki. Cleverly known as Butiki.

Studying at Kiira College Butiki reflected the Source of the Nile (Kiira). Kiira supplies electricity to Uganda & Kenya. It is the gateway to Eastern and Kenya. It is too a gateway to Kampala City and beyond.

Kiira College, in our times, was second to Mwiri College. This was so, because Mwiri merely mirroring for the Kyabazinga of Busoga, just like Kings College, Buddo mirrored the Buganda Kingdom[27]. Our Centre point used to be Wairaka Girls. Stop the script.

Kiira College Butiki was my preferred choice for secondary school development. It was actually after I had made the choice that I realised that my '*mythical cousin Owora Othieno*' formerly called Sunday was already an architect at the school. I have always wondered why you ever came to choose such a school that was hilly, the road impassable when it rained. The soils where red that could cake your white shirt and shorts all red.

---

[27] Ibid 18

I wonder how you managed to stay the course. At least for me, I joined Butiki at the same time Mr. Musanyana joined. He was a Mugwere and he studied with my Late Dad. He was one-eyed, but he was a no-nonsense headteacher.

By the time I joined Butiki, it was ungovernable, strikes where termly. In fact, it was widely known as the University of 'Strikes'. Mr. Musanyana came and changed all that. He started by expelling students even if its allegations were based on hearsay. He drew up his whip and his venom raided at the heart of any dissenting views.

I remember in my second year I was almost thrown out had it not been my *'mythical brother'* who sent an SOS from Nairobi City to pick up my Mum and Dad to come to the school and plead with Mr. Musanyana. It was because of my Mum as they had known each other so things cooled down. I was as lucky to have had a housemaster who was Mr. Osingili [RIP] from Rubongi who happened to have passed through the hands of my late Dad while he was a headmaster at Rubongi Primary School. He helped shape me by channelling my energy into extra curriculum activities.

That year I became the best actor in inter-house drama competition and our House took the trophy. As I moved on, I learned what my housemaster told me, and I joined various school clubs. I became Chairman of Science, Literacy club and was very active in in-house activities. In my third year I was made a Subsampler meaning I was now earmarked to become a school prefect, but alas! With *'mythical Musanyana'* at the helm, I was ruled out. So, I lost out in prefect-ship and became a commoner.

Now, back to my *'mythical friend'* GOOK, he arrived when I was in senior three. I did not know he came following the footsteps of the current Mayor of Pajwenda Town Council; 'Mayor Omwodo'.

Oh, my *'mythical friend'* Gook you looked too innocent like *'sleeping beauty'* on Vaseline label. I had thought I was your first player. You arrived loaded with all the material powers you could amass, thinking it would help you buy your way out. You were too loaded with this aura of the city living. You arrived at Kiira College Butiki and became what they termed at Butiki and as *'Empioko'*- meaning newcomer. You became a Republican I was already a Mulondian.

Looking back, I wonder how I came to know you. Ahh! There were the Pajwenda boys' one in Mulondo and another in Aggrey House. I suspect our first meet was because of a Pajwenda gentle giant by the name Othieno Obedo [RIP] who was a year ahead of me.

When you arrived, you looked like a Goliath: tall and slim as if underfed for Butiki life. I was short but ready for war. Remember the biblical 'Goliath' story it seemed that is how our relationship ended. I owned you and you became mine. You never failed to deliver. I became that cord of your obedience. I wonder how we hit that bond of friendship. Anyway, sometimes walls too have ears, so the saying goes.

I could not believe that for a long time you *'mythically hid'* behind my *'mythical back'*. I brought you up single-handed to view the world differently. I was like a single parent to you. However, that will be revisited another day.

I guess in terms of the *'mythical Olympic'* racing from Republic to Mulondo you were second to none. You know that the distance is one hundred meters apart. I remember one time you sprinted like the then *'mythical Carl Lewis'* to come and dive into my cassava. I wonder how your nose could smell my *'mythical cassava'* cooking on a stove one hundred metres away. Such was your smelling skills at its best.

Do you also remember that the *'mythical Republic House'* was next to the Mess [dining hall]. The moment the gong went you and other Republicans were the first troops to rush in and overpower 'mess' [dining hall] prefects to launch your forks into biggest potatoes or if it was meat day diving and forking the biggest meat

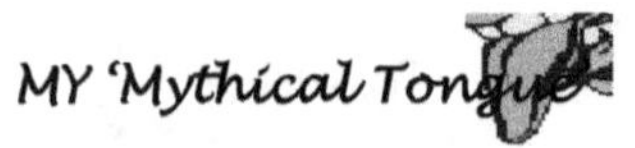

on the bone. Such were your architectural skills with a precision that became your best life skills.

I hope you remember when I kept reminding you that your hands were too short when launching them into your pockets and yet you were quick to launch your fork into the biggest potatoes or meat or sprinting into *'mythical Mulondo'* to dive at my *'mythical cassava'*. I kept *'mythical faith'* in you by *'mythically nagging'* you to strengthen and lengthen your *'mythical shorthands'*. In the end, it seems it worked for I *'mythically saw some results'*.

To be continued

JesseA

27

An Open Letter To My 'Mythical Learned Friend' GOOK The Lawyer.

28/05/2018

Dear Mythical Learned Friend GOOK the Lawyer

I have failed to understand why, when I left you in that KCB you kept creeping still inside my life, like some climbing plant that does not want to leave its prey like and an eagle with an eye on already captured meat by a creature below. You kept snaking around me, like an ensnared food captured by the python. Indeed, I became a sort of your '*mythical prey*'. I began thinking was it because of that '*mythical cassava*' at the '*mythical Butiki Hill*', that smell coming from the '*mythical Mulondo House*' that kept you '*mythically wanting*'.

I thought I had shaken you off my life, just like other OBs. I thought you would have moved on as you went to other pastures anew. You went into the '*mythical Kings College of Budo*' where the Baganda kings and queens are taught. I thought you would have looked at some of us as the subjects as you were being initiated into an object of the royalties. You went there and you started the process of learning how to become a lawyer and start the profession of using jargon Latin languages to win cases or fool the defence or prosecutors. You started this era with vigour. You went to this Higher school of learning they call the '*mythical*

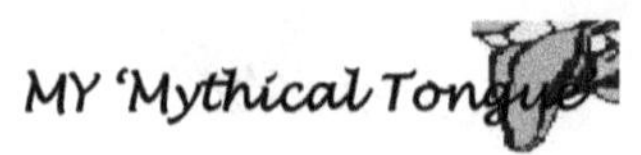

Makerere University'. You climbed into this ladder of attaining the Legal Bar studies to become a fully-fledged *'mythical lawyer'*. You graduated and learnt the tricks of luring and manipulating situations, so to say, as they are well known for that practise or malpractice. I became the first target of your manipulations and luring, using the common saying in the layman's circle.

You remember the *'mythical Mutungo Hill'* episode. You wanted to turn me into a *'mythical lawyer'* to represent your case. I had never ever gone to the Hill of higher learning to learn or study law, but you wanted to recruit me as your case lawyer, such was the scene. I told you I have never had any formal or any informal training or exposure into being a lawyer, let alone managing any case. You insisted that I climb into your car and go and represent you in some simple case that did not require any form of training but only common sense that you were aware is sometimes not common. You did not even check with me as to whether I had this common sense.

I was in a sense *'mythically kidnapped'* and ensnared into the belief that all would be okay at the end of the day. You insisted on driving me to the Mutungo Hill and delivered me to this court where there was this no no-sense female judge. I had never had this experience before, being arraigned in front of a female judge to make a representation case of a client whom I believe was my client now called Gook.

I was ill-prepared, *'mythically ill-trained, ill-advised, ill briefed and ill everything'* you can think of on this earth. You made me sit on the *'mythical lawyer's bench'* as your fence case lawyer. I was lost for words sitting on this bench to present a case for my supposedly client Gook, my *'mythical friend'*. I started sweating my *'mythical pants'* down that is if I had *'mythical pants'* at all. The handkerchief I had was full of *'mythical mucus'* and could not come to pull it out of my pocket to clean my sweaty face. Instead, I was forced to use my dusty hands to wipe my sweaty dusty face.

I was left with no options but to present the '*mythical case*'. My '*mythical body*' shivering in front of the female judge, my '*mythical voice*' breaking in syllables still I had to do this representation. Somehow, I had to compose myself and present this case as I was already a captive of my school sweetheart of KCB of Butiki. Whatever what 'sweetheart' meant. I stood up and stated my case as directed by my client. The defendant of the case had no prosecutors. One of the prosecutors who would have been me in the first place had already been ensnared into the opposition bench, in a sense, the soul bought out to win the case outright.

Having presented my case diligently I suppose, my '*mythical friend*' Gook had to now state his case clearly, he presented the alibi to the case in question. When asked about all the substantive shreds of evidence to enforce and back up his case, somehow, we had no further shreds of evidence to produce in this court. It looked like our case had failed the first hurdle. The '*mythical female judge*' had to postpone the case until all shreds of evidence were produced in court before she could hear this case any further. On top of that because of a one-sided case being presented, there was a need to have the prosecutors too, whom I could have been apart but now swallowed up. Such was my first day in this court and have had that initial circumcision experience of being the one wonder lawyer, I felt it deep inside to an extent that I did not need to be a lawyer but the law itself in this case again when it next comes in front of this tough-talking female judge.

To be continued

JesseA

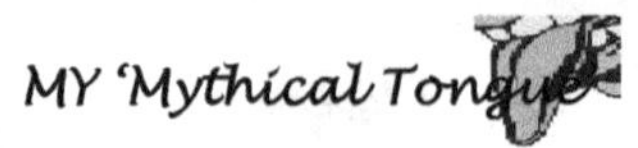

28

An open letter to my Mythical Sipi Choices.

11/07/2019

Hey!!! Mythical Sipi choices,

I tell you God works in mysterious ways. Why were you at the frontline when everyone had retreated into their trenches? How did you pick that courage to go to the battlefield unarmed, unaware dangers of dying in the battlefield?

You indeed gave me that straw that twigs to cling on in my hours of need; you wore your combats, unarmed and fought a war against the unpredictable. You were hands-on at that hour at that place ready to tackle the impossible. You turned what everyone saw as impossible, what everyone saw as a steep mountain to climb into a walkover.

Now on reflection, I sit down perplexed as to how you 'concomitantly' combated and single-handed won the 'Katanga war'. I tell you what you are such a genius. You are such a fresh air to breathe. When the *'mythical Katanga medal'* comes into production you will be the first one to wear it. I remember your ribs being kicked and shout of the call to eliminate the one ribbed combatant. You danced and swung like a biblical David and a Goliath thing fight, you know!!. You *'mythically dusted'* the dust, wore your war-torn camouflage and *'mythically moved on'*.

You saved an 'empire' without *'mythically firing any single shot'*. I wonder how you did it. How you built that courage. Anyway, I was told that; you used the tools you were given to rise up to be able to make a better decision than your forefathers. You vehemently read all those volumes and made the decisions to pick a stealth fighter. You chose your battles well and advanced with precision. Slowly but surely you did your bit. You showed others that you can use the acquired tools given to you in your lifetime to deliver a near to impossible, into reality. Present-day 'Katanga Region', being what it is; has been the *'mythical far-sightedness'* of a girl-child, my *'mythical Sipi Choices'*.

We are often told in dhopadhola saying that; *'inywolo ye wi'jaryo' [English speak - you should be born at least the two of you]*. It has proved the jopadhola saying right.

Anyway, I thank you in two folds you helped hold the Fort. I personally hold that especially dear, especially at the time, I was down and out when I was not sure whether I was going or coming, whether I was in or out. You helped me hold on to that straw, that twig that supported my sailing across the unknown abyss.

Here I am today looking at that milestone and being grateful. When I came back and explored the battlefields of the 'Katanga Region', you had conquered, it was such a joy. It lightened my heart, my spirits and my acumen. I was helpless but day in day out you looked out for me. You never winked when I coughed, snored, vomited or looked like a zombie. You were by the doorway checking on my welfare. I may have been a pain, but I was there because of you, because of that well-fought battle that you quietly and steadfastly managed to maneuverer it to the shores of the 'Katanga Region'.

You know what hold your nerves, fly your wings and be whatever you want to be all will be fine. No one should tell you that 'You Can not', cut off that 'Not' for 'You Can'.

To be continued

JesseA

29

An Open Letter To My Mythical Uncle My Best Friend Amunoni,

23/04/2019

Dear My Best friend

I just needed to shed some light on how we became best friends; you remember the *'mythical Nakivubo Post Office'*, those days. How time flies. Are those the days, one would call the good old days.

Those were the *'mythical good days'*. I can assure you that some of the secrets I will not mention it at all, as it will *'mythically shear'* of our true friendship. I will give you the highlights of and as whenever I landed at your *'mythical Nakivubo'* base when I was hungry from a three-month hideaway at boarding school. You held me and would give me the best meal for the day, I even wondered whether you had shares in that restaurant you every time took me to, as you would just take me and let the person in charge know I was yours to be served whatever I needed and you walked away.

You would even then quench my thirst with good cool Soda. You would then offer me the transport to Entebbe Town, sometimes you could let me hang around and we go off together. Those were the good days of bonding of that trust in *'mythical friendship'*. Sometimes there are the small things that make the big picture. These were one of those moments where picture collages are created.

Now I just needed a quick catch up of our recent interaction, you remember you quite intrigued me when you introduced me to that not so long-ago equation that over time it had even rusted in my brain. Remember you tried to teach me *'mythical BODMAS'*[28] or were it not. You tried to drill in my already tired *'mythical brain'* what *'mythical BODMAS'* equation means that; it is what they call Brackets, of Division, Multiplication, and Addition. You tried to turn your nephew pumpkin head into some mathematical and arithmetical genius. You remember we went through the ritual at a mathematical level to prove your point that reality and beauty of BODMAS is the ultimate equation that can sort and eradicate every human element at mathematical speak and at a *'mythical arithmetic level'*, to the point of reducing financial calculations to fit within the budgetary requirements.

You remember we had intense arguments that at a financial level your BODMAS equation can and should always compliment when at the divergence budgeting the unforeseen accounting and auditing would cater for even the hidden costings. Anyway, as for me, a social scientist, I had to give in to your scientifically and arithmetically proven equation, that is, the perfect element to solve every human mathematical need.

In your first lecture to me, I had even to google what this was all about, and this is what I came out with. It even confused me further.

"BODMAS RULE. BODMAS is an acronym and it stands for **B**racket, **O**f, **D**ivision, **M**ultiplication, **A**ddition and **S**ubtraction. In certain regions, PEDMAS (**P**arentheses, **E**xponents, **D**ivision, **M**ultiplication, **A**ddition and **S**ubtraction) is the synonym of BODMAS. It explains the order of operations to solve an expression."

---

28 https://www.google.com/search?q=BODMAS
https://www.google.com/search?q=BODMAS&sourceid=ie7&rls=com.microsoft:en-US&ie=utf8&oe=utf8

I was even more confused, so I had to go back to my friend google to ask another thing related to Mathematics and Arithmetic. It even produced flavours that my little brain could not dismember. *"Arithmetic[29] is to mathematics as spelling is to writing"*. It uses signs, symbols, and proofs and includes arithmetic, algebra, calculus, geometry, and trigonometry. The most obvious difference is that arithmetic is all about numbers and mathematics is all about theory.

I remain to be convinced in your next '*mythical lecture*' how 'creative accounting' too can fit-in within your '*mythical BODMAS model*'.

Thanks

Awaiting further lectures and recaps.

To be continued

JesseA

29 https://www.google.com/search?q=the+diffrence+between+matemtica+and+arithmatics&sourceid=ie7&rls=com.microsoft:en-US&ie=utf8&oe=utf8

30.

An Open Letter To My Mythical Nyenye The Pharmacist

02/06/2019

Saying Hi To my *'Mythical Nyenye'* the Pharmacist.

Praise be to my *'Mythical Nyenye'* the Pharmacist, you have made my *'mythical time'*, you indeed know your profession.

Time immemorial my *'Mythical Nyenye'* the pharmacist has always made *'mythical prescription'* to my *'mythical treatment'* and for my treatment too. She has always been on point when making prescription, prescribing as if there is no *'mythical tomorrow'*. It has always been the right doses at the right time in a good environment, for the right reason on that occasion that suits well.

However, over time my *'mythical pharmacist'* has sort of ignored the patient's wellbeing not even checking how the patient is doing. If you felt the medications you were prescribed was not working then why didn't you *'mythically engage'* the other pharmacist-gear-of-counselling me of the next course of your *'mythical actions'*. What happened?

I have never known that oceans dry and they do not accept new waters even when contaminated with residues; they still accept waters from the tributaries. So, my pharmacist why have you

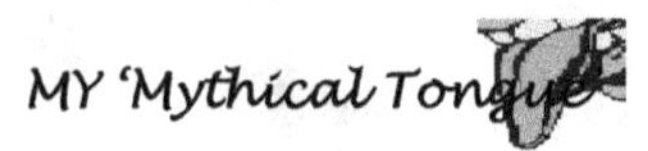

turned your face and back away from the old type style prescription.

Needless to say, the medications dried up the patient started having withdrawal symptoms that have now led to having withdrawal-syndrome to an extent that the patient started seeing and sourcing the medications from a *'mythical rogue pharmacist'* who was prescribing the wrong medication. My *'mythical pharmacist'*, what happened?

You were such a pharmacist who could be beckoned, called at short notice at any time of the day or night, because you had an open-door policy of meeting, seeing and dealing with your clients at short notice. You were always on point when prescribing and offering the doses and checking when it was over when to again make new prescriptions and supply. You never tweaked an eye when the patient wanted new doses whether he had taken more than normally prescribed dose because you trusted your patient so well.

Over time you have turned your back on the very patient you are meant to professionally look after. You have not even called your patient to check whether he needs to reconnect with you and your pharmacy. I may have a clue as to what happened, but I never believe in 'believing' in assumptions. Unless you come out and 'Out' it to me as to; why I no longer receive any prescription and supply from you.

My *'Mythical Nyenye'* the Pharmacist, you know what; I will *'mythically cling'* around here waiting for your response to my Open Letter to you, as my *'mythical withdraw symptoms'* and the syndrome anecdote has now reached a critical level whereby I may be forced to change a pharmacist and pharmacy altogether. But you know what, I will try to stick around as right now I have a new *'mythical 'Specialist Dr/Nurse Enid''*, who does not want me to come to your pharmacy for prescription and supply. She is a no-nonsense specialist that makes you very different.

But I leave that for another day. I will let you know how to go about that. Still, *'mythically cocooned'* in this corner hoping for your supply and support but then my *'Mythical Specialist Dr/Nurse Enid'* seems to be having a high stake on me right now, so I fear. As there is something about her that makes my blood coil the moment she speaks and appears. Even her shadows scare the life out of me. She acts like some *'Mythical Commanders'* I know, and suspect you also know them. This is just a whisper between us. But I still would love to be in your clinic anytime.

To be continued

JesseA

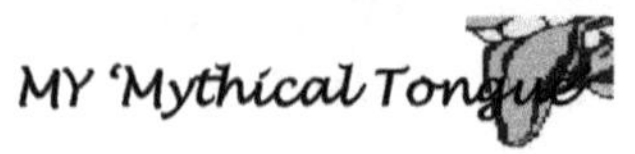

31

An Open Non-Disclosure Letter To My 'Mythical Brother Buluthi'

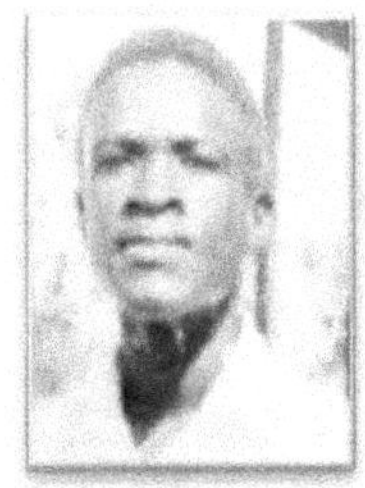

05/10/2019

Hey!! My *'Mythical Brother Buluthi'*,

I have had very painful thoughts, a virtual memory relapse, lapse and breakdown in putting this Open Letter to you, in order to understand why our tangents have been so divergent. This being my last Open Letter to all my *'mythical captures'* in this writeup shows how difficult it has been to pen this letter to you, but I have to, for ancestral reasons, I know the *'mythical ancestors'* would not be happy if I *'mythically caged in'* without passing on my thoughts to you. For as you know I still take advice from ancestral advisers still present, hence my letter to you.

You know how *'mythical ancestral advisors'* can be in touch with their *'mythical ancestral soothsayers'* and when they deliver advice just to let you know they will have had a very *'mythical nightly deep conversational'* moments that are bonded in the psyche.

You remember I came home twice and each time I felt the need to have a dialogue with you, my *'mythical brother Buluthi'*. I felt that each time you had an unexplained and developed indifference and animosity towards me. It appeared you never understood the purpose of my being there. I suspect it was at the behest of the *'mythical ancestors'*, who were trying to say something.

Seeing me, to you, I believe, it felt like I was occupying your rightful space, I suppose. In the end, we both missed the opportunity to hold each other as *'mythical brothers'* and make amends. As I always said, if you have any problem with me it is your problem and not mine. I cannot begin pursuing your agenda that I have no power and control over. Hence, I had to give you space to reflect on your deeds as I was not prepared to help you into that journey, which endgame I do not know.

Let me share with you my challenges when you were doing the *'mythical somersault'* with our dear *'mythical mum'* and *'mythical Sipi Choices'*, I was *'mythically down under'*, I was never sure whether I would be in or out. You challenged the very soul why *'Mythical Dad IOA'* bought that land for. You betrayed my *'Mythical Dad's legacy'*. You tried to create a two-tier system of the *'Mythical Them'*, and *'Mythical Us'*. The *"Mythical Us"* that was only themed around you and nobody else but you.

You tried to fracture, dismantle, obscure, the very existence of the *'mythical Broad-Church'' mythical family'* that had been carefully crafted, created and catered for by *'mythical Grandma Tolo'* and *'mythical Grandpa Ofano'*. This system has been passed on without a wink. At a stroke of your whims, you wanted to dismantle that existence and create an empire of selfishness that had never appeared in the vocabulary dictionary of our ancestors.

Your lust was a personal power ego that no one should look that side and think and say it is the right way. It is not the right way; others should look at it and say it is a no-go area. I am also too aware that the type of your *'mythical personal power ego'* can easily be sold to the *'mythically weak'*, the vulnerable at the point of need who cannot sit down, think, reflect and make sense as that is the directional approach to take; that can lead to detrimental effect.

Since we last engaged, you remember? When we sat down with you and *'mythical mum'* deep into the *'mythical mosquito-infested night'*, to chart a way forward and you were appealed to humble yourself and work for the good of the family. You shunned that and moved in the direction of your own personal and selfish ego and thoughts; that I may call your *'Mythical Power Trip'*. You tried to box some of us in your thoughts, but we were a bit cleverer than your thoughts.

I had never wanted to sound negative in a quest to bring out some of my own *'mythical personal issues'* to the fore. As I know my own *'mythical negativity'* towards you have to be unpacked, deranged, rearranged to make meaning as to why it is so. I have been pushed to spit out the pains in me, as it forms part of my own therapeutic sanity and healing to get out and move on for own personal existence.

I just hope before any next *'mythical engagement'*, for once you will have to look at your *'mythical self, diagonally, horizontally and vertically'* and then check yourself out how you really have to get out of that *'mythical shell'* and try and embrace others without spitting out any venomous toxin. You know what? People are very forgiving; you will be surprised how that can be. You will find yourself at the highest pedestal as a *'mythical prodigal son'*. For the sake of my beloved three *'mythical nieces'*, it is you to begin to move that *'mythical mountain'* you are entwined in; otherwise, the bandwagon is *'mythically rolling'* and is rolling very fast.

To be continued

JesseA

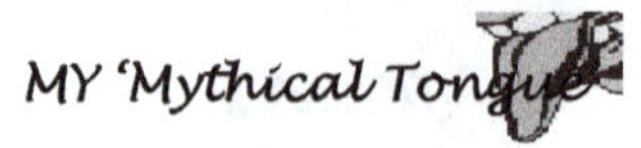

Epilogue

THE JOURNEY OF 'MYTHICAL WRITE-UP' BY JESSE ALECHO

02/06/2019

Following on from the *'mythical Introduction'* as I so painfully open up the epilogue with facts of my *'mythical illness'*, *'mythical pains'*, *'mythical denials'* but clinging on to *'mythical hope'*, I hope you will have followed why things happened in different sequences.

Looking back now, when I started writing up my *'mythical stories'* by using other *'mythical people'*, *'mythical scenarios'* to bring out what was in my *'mythical inner thoughts'*. Now on my own *'mythical reflections'*, I had *'mythically moved on'*. I had moved away from being me and becoming part of this *'mythical'* that I had to get in touch with to have a meaning and also to discuss what was going on and not going on in me.

I had psychologically entered a period of depression where illusions formed the core thinking of self. It gave me the satisfaction that I was there and yet my very existence had been blurred by these illusions whereby I was in an imaginary world and trying to walk through this maze to make sense of being me or having become somebody else. Life had *'mythically moved on'* and spiritually I was trying to play a *'mythical catch-up game'* to try and make sense of the world by creating a myth.

It was a *'mythical roller-coaster'* of thoughts that eventually developed putting things to be based on myths rather than being seen as real. However, the objects, the people I was attaching myself to or, rather, attaching my *'mythicals'* to, may have been illusory, but it reflected my inner thoughts of the cycle of things and issues that I was undergoing. Being hit with turbulence like in an aircraft and not knowing whether you can weather the storm and survive the storm, you cling to these emotions of thinking all is not there at this stage, all might be there or all can be lost in that split second.

I now realise how *'mythically painful'* to write about your pain as that pain is in the present and you have no control over it. It was funny that I could wake up do a write-up, type and broadcast it in a few hours. It sort of made sense of the urgency of the situation happening at that point in time. Hence, the *'mythical signs'* and putting something in place that may be untouchable but touchable too within a timeframe.

At the beginning of the *'mythical write-up'*, it was very difficult to put in writing my actual journey of the illness I was undergoing as I was aware that could easily be documented as the documentary facts were and are there.

However, the illusions, the myths around the illness and other emotions attached to it, unless I captured them at that stage and time, I would not remember in the next few minutes what I was thinking and what I wanted to write about, hence it would easily get lost in that maze of illusions, depressions, anxiety, name it.

As I continue to write *'mythically'*, I have found it a struggle to *'mythically sit down'* and write and document the *'mythical documented fact'*. But each time still these *'mythical illusions'*

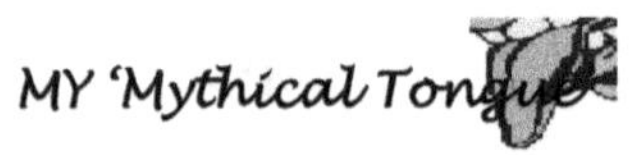

crop up and I write about them. It keeps me *'mythically sane'*. It keeps me moving. It still vibrates well with me in that *'mythical cocoon'*, I seem to have created. But it sounds safe in that way.

I have had discussions with several people who have supported and or questioned my *'mythical write-up'*, but I have on various occasions discussed with them the rationale of the write-up and the reason I have continued to do so; for I am still on this long journey to the unknown. One of the persons I discussed with having given him a sample of my *'mythical write-up'* and because he is a university student pursuing counselling psychology at Master's level and was writing up for his thesis is the one who braced me into the *'mythical reality'* that I equated all my write-up's to episodes of depression, denials. But here I am still writing and owning up that the truth may hurt but it is real. It is only holding the bull by its horns as the only way one can get out of the ditch. Am I anywhere near there? *'Mythically speaking'* God knows.

One person in particular about whom I will also write the *'mythicals'* is the one who had to call me telling me that people have been calling her asking about what is happening to me. I had to explain the reasons/rationale and she seemed to have understood. She gave me an anecdote of which I told her I will write about it and she found herself in the midst of the *'mythicals'*. This is how the story goes the journey I started with by kick-starting the first *'mythical write-up'* seems to be running riot in me.

While working with another colleague, a newly-qualified nurse by profession, I shared with her my brief write-up. She was taken aback and told me to read and watch movies by Professor Joseph Campbell. As she told me that whatever I was capturing in my *'mythical thoughts'* and write-up they are real and organic as is what the professor has documented. I have therefore had to do a brief watch and read on the signposted issues presented by Professor Joseph Campbell[30].

I have been overwhelmed and humbled how things happen in our subconscious and it is mirrored in our day-to-day thoughts and reality. So, I thank the convergence with the *'mythical colleague'*, the nurse whom the issue of the red microwave and radioactive remittance brought out excesses in our *'mythical conversation'* and brought the *'mythical disclosure'*.

The push to open up the hidden *'mythical wounds'* in me was compounded by my *'mythical brother'*, the Flight Engineer, who captured all my write-ups and told me to continue it in a book form.

I have had discussions with others who have, in a sense, given me *'mythical clues'* of the reasons for my *'mythical write-up'* as a sign of the conditions of *'mythical depression'* I have gone and/or is going through. In fact, I realise that this write-up may forever go on and on as it compounds various *'mythical segments'* of my past life, my present life, my future life and the unknown life. Such is the trend of what I am currently going through. Wrapping it and putting closure may be a long way off or it may be so near who knows.

To be continued

JesseA

---

[30] **Joseph Campbell** (March 26, 1904- October 30, 1987) was an American professor, writer, and orator best known for his work in the fields of comparative mythology and comparative religion. 8https://www.google.com/search?q=joseph+campbell&rlz=1C1GCEB_enGB859GB860&oq=joseph+campbell&aqs=chrome.0.0l6.5088j0j1&sourceid=chrome&ie=UTF-8

THE 'MYTHICAL ENDOSCOPY' THE REALITY

The procedure lasted for close to one hour. As there was a scar inside, hence it was painful and because they wanted to get out some tissue, they had to pinch some from the affected area. I could see the infection through the monitor. After that, I was told that I should get out of bed and to be not looking good.

Whereas others who came for similar endoscopy, others were being told all fine I was being told to wait in another room. I was specifically assigned to a nurse who would from now on look after my welfare. If I needed anything, I had to ring her or send a bleep and she would call me back. Such was the situation that I realised in the whole of **NHS**[31] whereby there were millions of people who were seeking treatment, I was specifically being assigned a nurse. If you imagine that scale of being personally assigned medical profession it showed the **NHS** was taking this case seriously.

I was assigned to a nurse from the Upper GI CNS TWR pathway.

[meaning I was under the care of Gastroenterology Intestinal, Cancer Nurse Specialist, of the Tactical Reconnaissance Wing] With a bleep and telephone number plus an email address.

Anyway, if you look at the abbreviation and if I was well educated, you could see that it meant more on the cancer pathway. So, I had actually been classified as a cancer patient without being directly told.

Anyway, I left after that I went back home too but knowing it was more than meet the eye.

---

31 **N**ational **H**ealth **S**ervice

i. **The *'Mythical Computerized Tomography'* (CT) scan 17th October 2017 for Thorax Abdomen Pelvis thrust contrast.**

Another appointment was arranged for the 17th October 2017 for CT. This is where I underwent a CT scan for Thorax, Abdomen, Pelvis thrust contrast to establish how far the disease had spread. By then I had not been told exactly what it was but was told it was under investigation to establish the actual disease they were narrowing on.

After I had attended the two appointments, I was sent another letter dated 20/10/2017 requiring me to attend the Gastroenterology outpatient's department.

ii. **The *'Mythical Result of Endoscopy'* and for CT scan for Thorax Abdomen Pelvis thrust contrast given on the 26/10/2017**

This appointment was for 10:30 am. This was a week after the CT scan which meant a total of three weeks to get the results and about a month since the GP had referred me. When I arrived at the clinic, I was taken inside and injected with a dye, to allow it to spread for better scanning. I was told to allow time for it to spread before they scanned me. That day I could not go to work as it involved more time at the hospital.

iii. ***The 'Mythical reality'* of the real result appointment date 26/10/2019 at 10.30am at the Gastroenterology outpatient's department.**

That morning I woke up carried my bags ready to go to work. I went for the appointment before proceeding to work.

At the appointment, I met with the consultant and my named nurse. The consultant asked me if I had come with anybody. I told him that I had not come with anyone. I settled down and that is when he told me that my diagnosis was "cancer".

However, they told me that at this moment they could establish the extent of the disease until they carried out other tests to that effect.

Was it a bombshell for me? I have tried to look back and cannot look at or have that experience of what real feeling it was. This may further explain the aspects of denials, by creating shockproof self to continue moving on. The Consultant asked me if I had made an appointment for the PET-scan but I told him that I was having difficulty doing so though I received a letter and phone call messages.

The named nurse supported me after the consultation, and she rang the PET-scan department and an appointment was booked. Moreover, it was just after my next appointment to meet the oncologist consultants.

iv. The *'Mythical reality'* of explaining to people how I felt when it involved the disclosure of the 'C'-word

When I tell people about my diagnosis what they tend to ask is how I felt when there was this bombshell of being told you had the 'C' word that no one wants to mention and scared of. I have reflected on it and realised that it could have affected me and subdued me.

When faced with a crash, let's say you are on a head-on collision with another vehicle, what would be ones thought process in that mad moment. Quite often the words that come out in cases of danger is Oh My God! In Jopadhola's speak! In a mother tongue, we cry out loud' Oh mama yee! Means ohh! My mother! Basically, it is your *'mythical mother'* who has produced you and you feel like disappearing back into her tummy. I believe this is where my first thoughts collapsed *'mythically speaking'*, on my *'mythical mother's''* lap and trying to rush back into her *'mythical tummy'* as if I never had anything said.

My first thought went to my elderly mother whom I was concerned about. I felt that she is elderly and has buried many of my siblings and my son included. I felt I would not like that; my death to be her point of demise on this earth. I could not imagine how she would hold it together when I passed away and saw my body being interred before hers.

It went through my mind as this similar situation happened in the family before where my '*mythical grandmother Tolo*', buried her grandson and immediately another of her other sister in law passed away there and then. She could not hold anymore her heart gave way and she passed on.

Another thing that left me feeling maybe lack of empathy on myself and pounding with self-pity of passing on was that eight months down the line I lost my son of 26 years of age when I found him dead in bed, at his flat. So, who am I who has reached my end-of-life stage should continue thinking of being alive? It did not make sense that my life was more important than the one I have just buried. I got my workbag ragged but determined that life was to go on. I left for work. At work, I emailed my manager who was concerned about many phone contacts and wanting to know what was wrong. I had told her I did not know what it was as they were carrying out investigations. I then told my line-manager that I had been diagnosed with cancer and she told me that I should tell her anytime how I feel. Reflecting back, I believe I was a walking Zombie but pretending to still be having some degree of sanity.

v. The '*mythical idea*' of disclosure to the immediate family and management of the information

I could not get around telling my children as they were also undergoing other issues that are hard to address here.

Disclosure to my wife. I went home after work and then I had to break the news to my wife. I then let the C-word out of the bag to her.

How she reacted or received the information is something I cannot say or would not know as people take news differently. Throughout my treatment and after I have read extensively and I now realise that it is difficult to get people's true feelings and how they react to different situations differently.

Disclosure to my brother, formerly known as Seven-Thirty. I

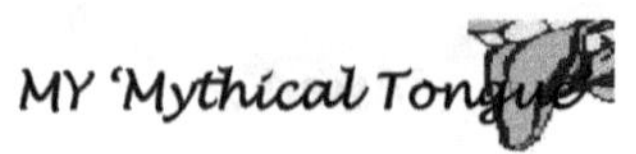

pondered as to when I would inform him, but I had to wait for some selling point when I could let him know what the situation was. This was only done after I had received all the information from the clinicians and when I knew the type of treatment I was to undergo and what the expected result was to be and when the treatment was to begin.

Disclosure to my '*mythical son*' famously known as Arnie. I could not disclose to him, for various reasons that I will explain later in the write-up.

Disclosure to my *'mythical son'* currently known as Kaio X R '01 I also could not disclose to him at this point in time for various reason I will explain in the later write-up.

vi. The *'Mythical reality'* of meeting the Oncologist Consultant at the Oncology out-patients 03/11/2017.

I had an appointment arranged to now formally meet the oncologist who was going to work with me. I met with the oncology team that included my chemotherapy and radiotherapy oncologist consultants plus now I was again given another named new nurse whom I could call at short notice in case of need.

The two consultants said I needed further scan, blood and kidney analysis to establish the course of treatment. *EDTA*[32] *[EDTA is used extensively in the analysis of blood. It is an anticoagulant for blood samples for CBC/FBEs, where the EDTA chelates the calcium present in the blood specimen, arresting the coagulation process and preserving blood cell morphology*]

However, they could not yet begin treatment as they were not sure if the infection had spread beyond or not hence the need for the PET-scan, because there was a shadow by around the heart area. They needed to make sure it had nothing to do with it had

32 https://www.google.com/search?rls=com.microsoft:en-US&q=EDTA https://www.google.com/search?rls=com.microsoft:en-US&q=EDTA+%5BEDTA+is+used+extensively+in+the+analysis+of+blood.+It+is+an+anticoagulant+for+blood+samples+for+CBC/FBs,+where+the+EDTA+chelates+the+calcium+present+in+the+blood+specimen,+arresting+the+coagulation+process+and+preserving+blood+cell+morphology&spell=1&sa=X&ved=0ahUKEwjBxsrY__jjAhXKiVwKHVUgAdAQBQguKAA&biw=1280&bih=657

spread outside the areas of containment.

On the day of the PET-scan I was told that I shouldn't eat or eat any sweets but to drink as much water as possible. I went for the scan and I was injected with a radioactive substance to supply them to map the areas of infections. They checked my sugar levels. Prior to this scan, I had to do blood tests. The PET-scan normally lasts for approximately 45 minutes but it is the preparation that takes a lot longer. I was injected with a radioactive material that should take effect after 45 minutes before being taken to the scan. After the scan, I was not supposed to be near children or pregnant women.

After this, I was told to wait a week before seeing my consultant.

vii. The *'mythical reality'* of meeting the Oncology consultant 10/11/2017 for the result of PET-scan and blood test result.

After that, I had to meet with my consultants who now agreed to the course of treatment for both chemo and radiotherapy. I was told that I would undergo a 5 to 6 course of chemotherapy and 30 sessions of radiotherapy. I was told both would run concurrently.

The diagnosis was thus: - Squamous cell carcinoma of the oesophagus 32 and 38 cm T4N2MO with aortopulmonary window node? significance. I was told for now they were trying to go for an outright cure though they would not guarantee me that in 15 years or so it will not reappear. I was also told about my appearance that would change. My consultant told me I would or may end up as dark as a Mali. She was very pleasant. She told me that I might lose hair. She listed to me all the side-effects I may experience name it? It was there on the list. I was told that she was the first medical professional who would tell me not to diet but eat as the effect of medicine would take its toll. I was told that the medication they were going to treat me on Cisplatin and Capecitabine.

10/11/2017 appointment also with the chemotherapy department to see how the treatment was to begin. At the same time, I was to do blood tests that would allow them to assess as to the quantity and type of medicine they should mix for my treatment.

I was given an appointment to go and discuss my chemotherapy at the clinic as things would go on the same day. I went up to the chemotherapy wing and discussed with lovely nurses who were going to take care of me for the next six months or so.

The chemotherapy was to run every 21 days followed by tablets in between.

I met both the chemotherapy oncologist and radiotherapy consultant who agreed with the course of treatment to begin. I signed the consent form to agree for the treatment to begin as they had recommended.

viii. The '*Mythical Journey*' of Chemotherapy

14/11/2017 Chemotherapy began

On the day of the beginning of the treatment, I went with my wife to begin the long journey to chemotherapy. I was taken in they did the normal process of the drill of being given a wrist band, hospital gown and putting in the equipment to begin giving me the treatment via venous access.

The treatment was to last 6 hours on the trot. This meant 2 hours was for first hydration IV, and then 2 hours of actual chemo treatment, then the last two hours was again of rehydration. So, as I went at 10.00 am, I left the clinic at five.

On my first day, I could see people I came with were living earlier than me. People who came later could just come in for an hour or two. I later, learnt that each person's treatment was different, however, similar the diagnosis might be. On a first day it was done I was ready to go I felt nothing really after the course of the doze. After which I was given steroids and medication to take whenever I felt like vomiting. I was given tablets to take for the next 21 days in the morning and evening pacing it 10 hours apart.

The next day I work up and went off to work feeling normal. It was in the course of the week when I started feeling weird. So, one day I had to inform the manager that I had to leave at lunchtime.

I had now to disclose to some of my colleagues about my diagnosis and illness rather than them seeing changes in me and not understanding what is going on. Therefore, I informed a couple of them and they were extraordinarily supportive.

This was going to be very painful, but I had to disclosure to my *'mythical son'* famously called Arnie. My son, since after the death of his brother, had a mental breakdown. He struggled throughout the time we came back from Uganda following the burial. So, during the time I was being diagnosed, he was also undergoing his own crisis. By the time I was diagnosed he had to be hospitalised too. He was discharged on the same day I had my first chemotherapy. It was so painful for me. When I came back home from the clinic, he was back home. I had first to ensure he was stable.

Over the weekend I got a car, we went around up to Brixton and did some shopping. We came back to Streatham all to try to see if he was ready to receive the news. It was also to get both him and his brother to blend as a lot of water had flowed under the bridge during the instability period.

After two weeks when I felt that my *'mythical son Arnie'* was now stable enough, I called him into my bedroom and confided in him what I was undergoing and reassured him the medical professionals were on top of things. I then asked him if it was okay for me to also disclose to his *'mythical brother'* currently known as Kaio X R '01. He told me not to do so yet. I listened to him and left it at that.

I had also to disclose to my *'mythical brother'* formerly known as Seven-thirty that same weekend. I called him and we met at our local pub. We had a discussion and disclosed to him what I was undergoing, the diagnosis and treatment. We then agreed that he would come in the next round of chemotherapy treatment. He assured me that at least we are in a country where the facilities are available. He just asked me to be strong, hold it and get on with the treatment and get better is all he can wish for.

Before my second chemo treatment, I had now to get through another hurdle to inform my *'mythical son'* currently known as Kaio X R '01. I knew it was not going to be easy for him, so I had to think hard how to deal with it. What I did was the Friday before my next course of treatment I had to go to his school and met the school administration and they had been supportive during the time when he lost his brother. So, I arranged a meeting with them. I disclosed to them about my ailment, the treatment I was undergoing and the prognosis. I wanted them to continue supporting him as I was going to let him know over the weekend.

So, over the weekend, I called him into the room, and we discussed my illness and what the expected outcome was. I then invited him to come to the hospital after school to the chemo ward so that he sees the process and then go back home together. I do not know how he felt but he was calm about it.

One time in the night, some form of thing came into my mind and was telling me to read Biblical Matthew Chapter 7. I wondered what this was all about. I had to get back as I was awake, opened my smartphone and read the whole of chapter 7. I did not know why it came to my mind. The only thing I could relate to was that my late grandfather Ofano when he nicknamed his son Levi as Matayo.

On the 12/12/2017, I had a second chemo course. My brother came along, and we were there chatting as the treatment was taking its course. Eventually later, after my son had finished school, he joined us and sat there watching the processes. My brother then left us and shortly after that after the treatment course, we left together for home.

After this, I had to book for my two sons to go to their auntie in Sweden for Christmas so that they could bond and because I felt that I did not want them to have a Christmas that would have no meaning to them following what had gone under the bridge.

ix. An open disclosure to my *'mythical cousin Dr Oteki'*

When I realised I was sinking deep in the sand in the treatment and illness taking its toll, I had to disclose to my *'mythical cousin'*, and ask him for advice whether I should disclose to home people as information can get out of hand and moves in all directions that we may have no control over. He is my refection hence anything to do with the home front and inside the idea of how to deal with situations, I discussed with him for he is second to none in the field of reflectional study.

However, he assured me that the most important thing was for me to undergo the treatment and get better. I should not bother getting out information to other people, as it would just stress me and others too. I listened to his advice and kept the disclosure to the very minimum.

My real relationship with the one I look like my twin my *'mythical cousin Dr Oteki'* dates quite back as we are almost closely matched in terms of age group structure. He has been instrumental in my wellbeing and in ensuring that he gave me rightful advice whenever I needed it. He will tell me things the way they are and not try to beat about the bush. Quite often, he would volunteer it without even me opening my mouth. When I am feeling low and on the 'hard rock' he knows and covers my back so well. He is indeed my confidant I would say in every way, like or form.

x. A disclosure to My *'mythical uncle Amunoni'*

The only other person I confided in was my *'mythical uncle Amunoni'* as he was involved in the welfare of my mother and helps in supporting me run some projects in Uganda. As I had stopped work and there was going to be no money stream, he would get concerned. Therefore, I had to disclosure to him so that he would be prepared to support me. He too told me to get on with the treatment and not waste my time and energy worrying about letting other people in the know. He would keep me safe.

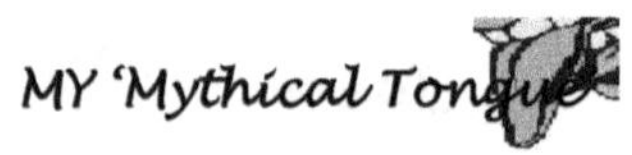

xi. **Second *'Mythical PET-scan Review'***

On the 08/12/2017 met with the oncologist to review how the first course to chemo went. I was feeling weak, lethargic, limbs kept giving way and muscles twitching. The consultants had to book me in for another PET-scan to establish the treatment was working and to check if the suspicion of and outside shadow had anything to do with cancer.

xii. ***My 'Mythical psychological visit to O'busy'***

On the 9/12/2017 I booked my membership car and moved around especially to visit my *'mythical niece O'busy'* for she had brought to the world another gran. I knew I needed to do this quickly as the treatment was taking its toll. As I was told, my physical and emotional being would change so I needed to do ward rounds so that people would not be suspicious if I disappeared from social circulation. I had a good time and discussed things close to my diagnosis, but I did not disclose to her. I remember discussing the Manuka honey to support with taste, that the consultant had recommended and here it was; she had it and I tasted it.

xiii. **Visiting the *'mythical LALiz family'***

From My *'mythical Obusy's'* we proceeded to see the other part of Croydon relatives the parents to my *'mythical son's Kaio X R '01 confidant'*. I knew that this family would, over time, support me and my son if he needed peer support and when rough times struck, he had a fallback position. Therefore, I had to get to them to disguise my illness under the pretext of ordinary visitation. We chatted, ate and left then left to get back home. At this moment, I felt that, at least, as far as social circles were concerned, I had, sort of, covered the track so that as the treatment and sickness were taking its toll, people would not be too suspicious.

xiv. ***'Mythical end of a curtain at RBKC'***

On the 19/12/2017 I had to call it a day and close the chapter when I realised that it was getting increasingly difficult for me to deliver service and at the same time being on treatment. I realised it was taking its toll. Fatigue, tiredness vomiting name it was having a field day. I had to leave work with the RBKC where I was working with the Grenfell residents to support those getting alternative accommodations.

xv. **Below are the sentimental card messages that my colleagues wrote to me and sent me an M&S voucher for £50. It was so touching to know colleagues cared.**

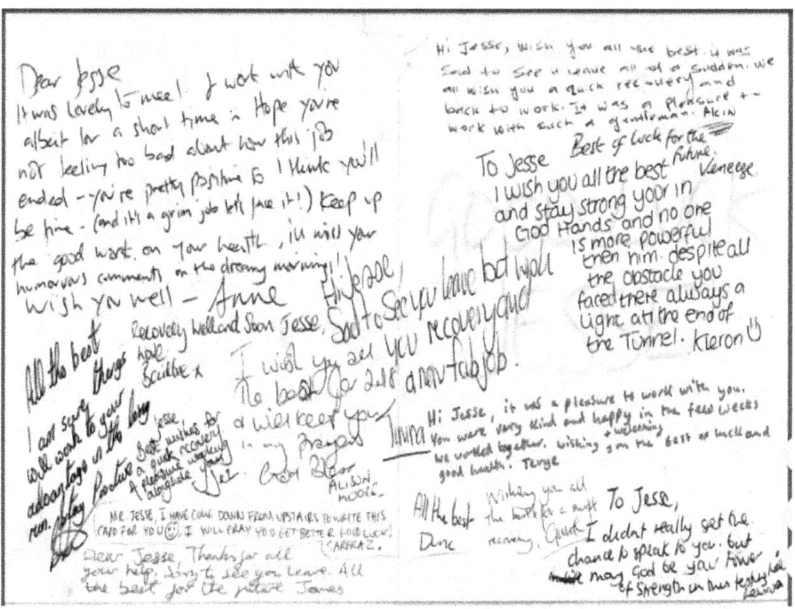

xvi. **On the 27/12/2017 PET-SCAN @10.30AM.**

I was booked in to check after two chemo cycle whether it had captured the cancerous cells. I underwent similar routing as the first scan.

xvii.

Second '*Mythical Result of the PET-scan*'

On the 05/01/2018, I met both consultants for chemo and radiotherapy to get the results of the PET-scan. I was shown the results via the computer. Initially, the cancerous area was yellow over a wide area. But this result showed that there was no trace of the yellow area all was red. The consultant told me it showed a positive response to the treatment and therefore they would go ahead with combined chemo and radiotherapy.

xviii. *'Mythical disclosure'* to Cousin Sister and My In-law Both Doctors Based in Canada Drs The Mythical Mus'.

After this, I had to give a call to my other team of the disclosures. This was to my *'mythical cousin'* and my in-law - both medical doctors based in Canada Drs The Mus'.

When I disclosed to them, it was heartbreaking when they received the information. In fact, they had wanted to fly straight to London to be by my side. However, I had to assure them that, other than the side-effects of the treatment, I was okay. I told them I would get by as best I could.

I know how whenever you mention to someone on the phone especially when they are not seeing you and you mention the word 'Cee'. I believe when they heard from me, they thought it was terminal. They asked what they could do to support me. I reassured them that other than the illness and leaving work, for now, all was okay though it may be tough times ahead. I had to scan the medical information and sent to them so that they could understand the illness, medication and anything else they could learn from it.

At this point, because they are all medical professionals, they read and understood everything I sent them. From then on, they could ring to check how I was. From time to time I also gave them updates about my situation.

xix. *'Mythical CT scan'* at Royal Marsden Hospital

Booked for CT scan to Royal Marsden Hospital to begin radiotherapy on the 29/01/2018. So, I went to Royal Marsden Hospital in Sutton on the day and I was put through the machine to map out the area the radiotherapy was supposed to be administered. After that, it was marked as a tattoo and was told to report on the 29/01/2018.

On the 29th it was not meant to be as I missed my chemo due to flu and, as a result, they could not do the concurrent radiotherapy hence it was postponed.

xx. **Disclosure to My '*mythical friend GeofB*'**

I invited my '*mythical friend GeofB*' a Zambian and I disclosed to him what I was undergoing, and he reassured me of the need to be strong and undergo the treatment all would be fine. He then disclosed to me that ten years ago he was also diagnosed with skin cancer on his legs and he had to undergo both chemo and radiotherapy and since he has been fine. So, he gave me the reassurance of being able to overcome, based on my prognosis. He also disclosed to me that he had another friend who had just undergone both treatments for prostate cancer and there was the chance that he would be fine at the end of it. From then on, he has supported me to-date to discuss and look at anything positively. We often crack jokes and say sometimes we just need a '*mythical laugh*' and not take life too seriously '*mythically speak*'.

xxi. **Disclosure to my '*Mythical Vicar*' of the Holy Redeemer Church**

I had to make an appointment to see my vicar. I had to disclose for the church had been very helpful to us as a family. On the day I went to see my vicar, I broke the news to him. And he told me we should read Psalm 27 together. Thereafter, he reassured me of his personal and church support. He asked me what part of the Holy Bible I wanted to read. I told him that sometime back I was in the dreams that instructed me to read Matthew 7. He then asked me which part I was interested in. I replied that I did not have any preference as I had read it but failed to get the gist of it. So, we read the whole of Matthew 7. Then we said the grace and we parted company.

From then on, the vicar kept on ringing me and coming home to check on me. I also kept on updating him on how I felt and at what level I was with the treatment.

xxii. Booked for CT scan at the Royal Marsden to begin radiotherapy on the 29/01/2018.

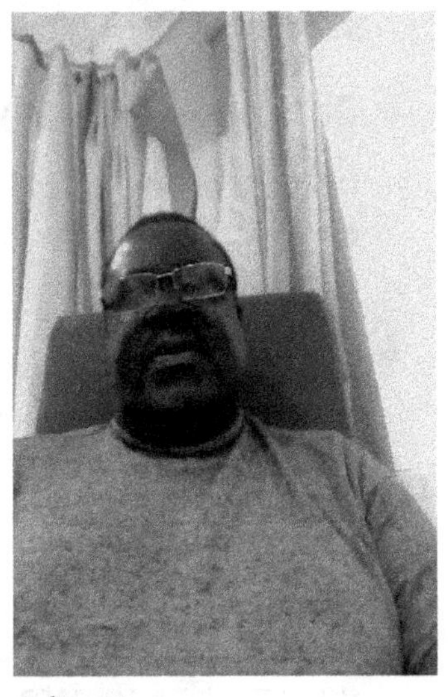

xxiii. ***'Mythical meeting'* with the Consultant**

2/02/2018 meeting with chemo consultant. As I was meant to have had another 4th course of chemo but due to flu and low blood cells, it was put off by another week or so to monitor. I was put on Granulocyte-colony stimulating factor (G-CSF). I was also injecting my tummy for five days before being reviewed again to see if I could be ready for the next course of chemo treatment.

09/02/2018, I met chemo oncologist to review whether could go back into treatment. She was satisfied and I was booked in for the 3rd chemo treatment to take place on the 13/02/2018.

xxiv. **6th January/2018. Reflection as I was doing some *'Mythical write-up'*. A day before my birthday.**

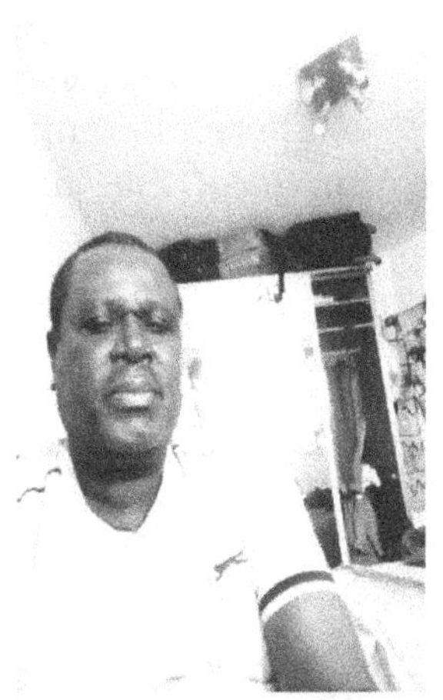

xxv. **9th January-2018 more reflections as I was doing my *'mythical write-up'* and telling lies to my *'mythical lawyer GOOK'***

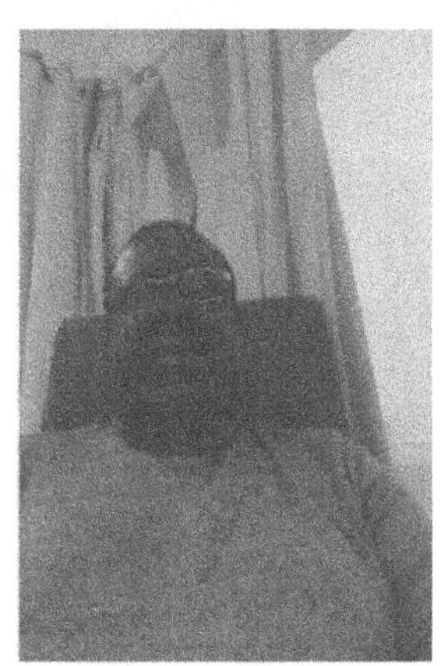

xxvi. ***'Mythical Birthday Bash'* for my gran Issy of my *'mythical niece O'busy'***

On the 13/01/2018 my *'mythical niece O'busy'* had a birthday bash for my gran *'mythical Issy'* who had made one year born on the same day as me On the 7th of January. I met so many relatives and chatted life away. On that day, I also came face to face with my *'mythical Miss-N'* with my future IOA in replacement. He came by me and we had quite a good friendly chat and he made my day. For once I had it whispered into my ears that he was the future. I cowed into '*mythical me*' as I was in the '*mythical birthday*' of my '*mythical Issy*'.

xxvii. **Third Chemotherapy - 16th /01/2018**

I attended my 3rd Chemo. By then the body was like wired through some electric circuits. Acting very funny limps doing all sorts of destruction on my life. This birthday celebration meant a lot to me.

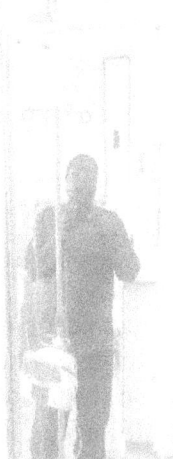

xxviii. **Reflection as I was doing some '*Mythical write-up*'.**

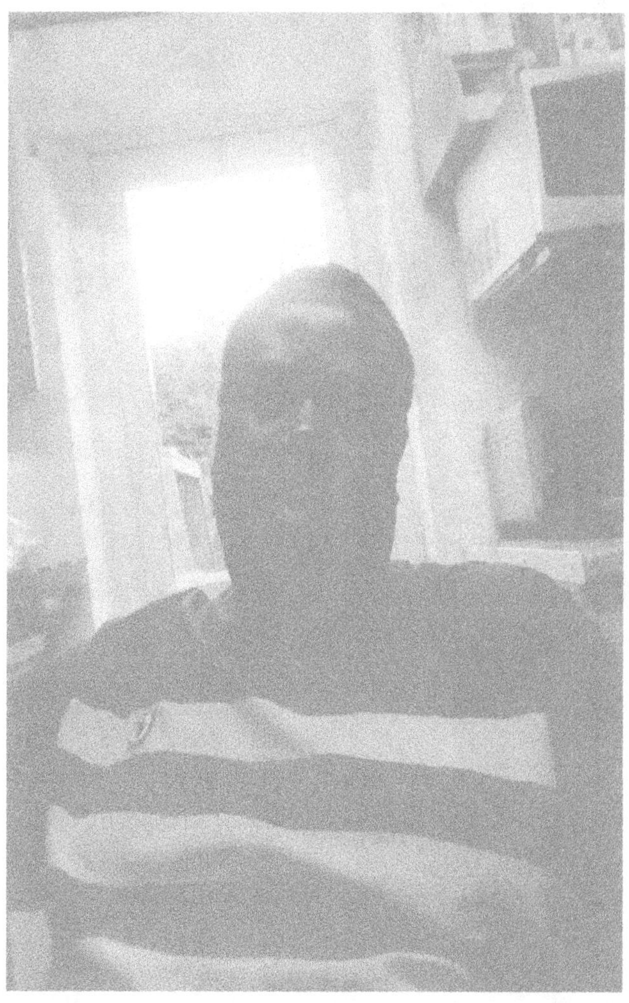

xxix. **13/02/2018 4th Chemo day**

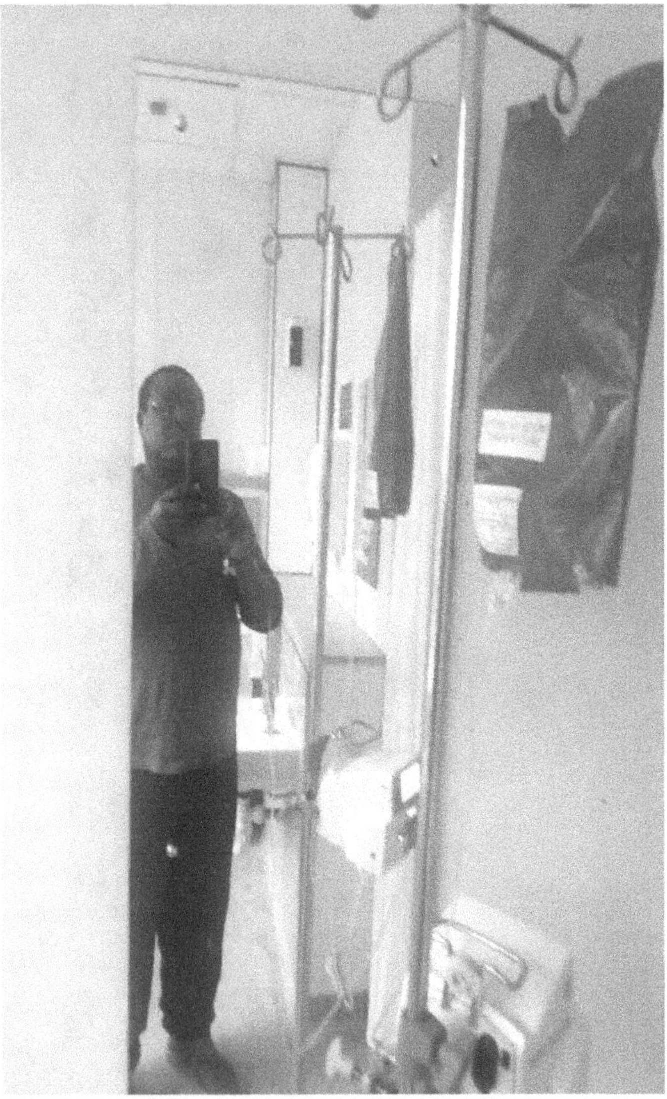

xxx. 6/03/2018, 5th and last of the MOT chemo day the last chemotherapy

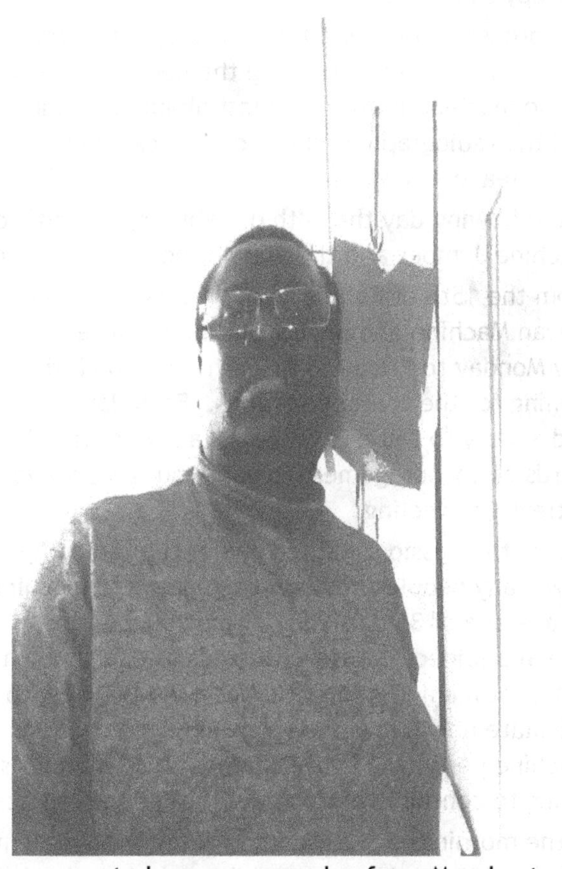

Radiotherapy was to happen every day from Monday to Friday, five days a week for thirty sessions. I started on radiotherapy on the 13th of February 2018, as the chemo had been delayed. I reported for the treatment at 9.30 am to begin the process. The machine I used was Hawthorn on that day. The process involved getting off my clothes and getting into the hospital gown, going through the ritual of name, date of birth, address and then, being given a wrist label carrying my names, date of birth, hospital and NHS reference number, then taken into the radiotherapy room. The RN's then go through the rituals of confirming my name, date of birth my physical address. On the radiotherapy room radiographers then began the process of aligning me to the required area where the focus of the therapy should be focused on.

The processes once set the radiographers then leave the room and the machines start doing the needful. The whole process of the machine movements last about ten minutes then stops, and the radiographers then come back and lower the bed for me to leave.

The following day the 14th of February, I used a different machine Juniper and the appointment was for 1.40 pm.

From the 15th of February for 11 sessions, I was attached to Rowan Machine and my appointments were for 10.30 am each day Monday to Friday. I made friends to all those who were coming for the therapy sessions. Each day any I met or saw had a story to tell each other. Each one was giving the other words of encouragement even if you saw how your other patient was feeling.

During this session, I asked one of the radiographers roughly how many people they saw each day on a machine. I was told an average of 35 patients per machine per day. Now imagine patients joined at different levels as each person requires different many sessions. It was mind-boggling to try and calculate how many patients were seen by RHM per day per machine per year. I gave thumbs up to them. As they were trying to contain what you would see as an epidemic.

In the mornings as I appeared for my appointments, it was quite disheartening to see children being wheeled into the radiotherapy rooms to undergo the treatment. I silently and internally asked myself if an illness may be a result of bad deeds, then what would this child have done at this early stage to deserve this. I looked at myself inwardly and lamented that at least at my age I had done all types of things good or bad, on this earth and maybe I deserve such illness but not an innocent child. But again, having such reflections made me stronger as an illness has nothing to do with bad deeds, but it is just what it is. Someone has to get sick and that includes me and a child as well, for we are humans still breeding and have to undergo certain pains in life.

My fourteenth session was on the 02/03/2018 at 8.50 am at Hawthorn Machine.

My fifteenth session was on Rowan Machine at 9.40 am and thereafter I met with the consultant at 10.15 am to review the treatment. At this stage then I was prescribed Food supplements as could no longer have food or drink intake and appetite was down to zero. Bodyweight was falling.

On the 6th of March was my sixteenth Radiotherapy session and it was adjusted to be at Hawthorn machine at 8.40 am because that day I had to combine it with the last chemotherapy treatment at St George's University Hospital. Having attended the radiotherapy at RMH I then preceded to St George's University Hospital for the last dose of chemo.

From the 7th until the 18th March I used the Rowan Machine those were for 8 sessions.

xxxi. Tuesday 6th March 2018. 5th and last day of Chemotherapy at St Georges University Hospital.

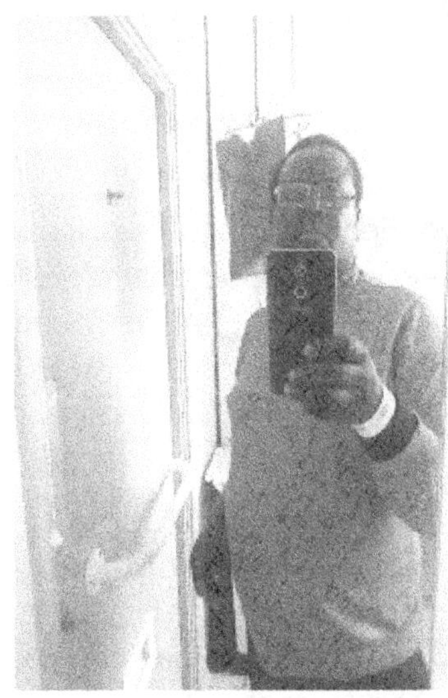

xxxii. The *'Mythical Journey of Radiotherapy Treatment'* that was to last for thirty sessions.

I started on radiotherapy on the 13th of February 2018, as the chemo had been delayed. I reported for the treatment at 9.30 am to begin the process. The machine I used was Hawthorn on that day. The process involved getting off my clothes and getting into the hospital gown, going through the ritual of name, date of birth, address and then being given a wrist label carrying my names, date of birth, hospital and NHS reference number and, finally, being taken into the radiotherapy room. The RN's then went through the usual rituals of confirming my name, date of birth my physical address. On the radiotherapy room radiographers then began the process of aligning me to the required area where the focus of the therapy would be focused on.

Once the process was set, the radiographers left the room and the machines started doing the needful. The whole process of the machine movements last about ten minutes then stop. The radiographers then come back and lower the bed for me to leave.

The following day the 14th of February, I used a different machine, Juniper, and the appointment was for 13.40 hours.

From the 15th of February for 11 sessions, I was attached to Rowan Machine and my appointments were for 10.30 hours each day Monday to Friday. I made friends with all those who were coming for the therapy sessions. Each day whenever I met or saw any of them, we had a story to share. Each one was giving the other words of encouragement even if you saw how the other patient was feeling.

During this session, I asked one of the radiographers roughly how many people they saw each day on a machine. I was told an average of 35 patients per machine per day. Now imagine patients joined at different levels as each person requires different many sessions. It was mind-boggling to try and calculate how many patients were seen by RHM per day per machine per year. I gave thumbs up to them because, to me, they were trying to contain what would be seen as an epidemic.

In the mornings as I appeared for my appointments, it was quite disheartening to see children being wheeled into the radiotherapy rooms to undergo the treatment. I silently and asked myself if an illness might be a result of bad deeds, then what would this child have done at this early stage to deserve this? I looked at myself inwardly and lamented that, at least, at my age, I had done all types of things good or bad, on this earth and maybe I deserved such illness but not an innocent child.

But then again, having such reflections made me stronger as an illness had nothing to do with bad deeds, but just what it was. Someone has to get sick and that includes me and a child as well, for we are humans still breeding and have to undergo certain pains in life.

My fourteenth session was on the 02/03/2018 at 8.50 am at Hawthorn Machine.

My fifteenth session was on Rowan Machine at 9.40 am and thereafter I met with the consultant at 10.15 am to review the treatment. At this stage then I was prescribed food supplements as I could no longer have food or drink intake and appetite was down to zero. Bodyweight was falling.

6th of March saw my 16th Radiotherapy session and it was adjusted to be at Hawthorn machine at 8.40 am because that day I had to combine it with the last chemotherapy treatment at St George's University Hospital. Having attended the radiotherapy at RMH I then proceeded to St George's University Hospital for the last dose of chemo.

From the 7th until the 18th I used the Rowan Machine. Those were altogether 8 sessions.

xxxiii. The '*Mythical Journey*' from Sutton to 125-Second Avenue.

On 9th March after I had finished my 19 sessions. The body was too weak, and I was almost no longer coping. However, that day being Friday I felt I needed to venture to East London to my brother's place. I was feeling quite awful, but I was determined to make the journey somehow. I got into the train up to Manor Park. However, the trip was tiring. I was exhausted as the train journey took around 2 hours. To move from the station to my brother's house took me close to one-and-a-half hours what would normally just take me 15 minutes.

I kept on stopping on the way to catch my breath, get a breathe. Eventually, I arrived and knocked on his door. He was inside and he opened the door. He welcomed me and sat me in the lounge. He asked me if I wanted anything to eat. The only thing I told him was that I just needed to sleep. He then showed me a bed to lie in. When I woke up, I dragged myself down to the lounge. He gave me some food. We had a bit of a chat. He then asked me if he should drop me home. I told him I had no energy to get around again.

I was really very weak, exhausted, fatigued, name it. I slept there overnight. Next day the 10th of March 2018, lunch was prepared and then after that, my brother decided to drop me back home.

The one reflection about this visit to me was like I had lost hope, I had given up. I equated it to when my late brother came to my house and all he wanted was to sleep. He slept up to around 8.00 pm and had encouraged him to stay overnight as he couldn't drive when he was that weak. It was towards his last days on earth. What he told me when he wanted to go back home was about one-word 'Dignity'. So, when my brother was dropping me home that word my late brother told me 'Dignity' stayed in my psyche and remains so to this day.

xxxiv. On the 12th of March 2018,

I resumed my move to begin the 20th session of radiotherapy. I went on up to Friday the 16th when I did my 24th radiotherapy session.

The weekend followed I could hardly move out of bed and by then the weather was so vicious and nasty to venture outside. On the 19th of March 2018, I had to be admitted in hospital as a result of dehydration, no eating and heavy loss of weight. By the time I was admitted I had lost 13 kilograms of body weight. That morning I went normally for my daily radiotherapy. I could hardly make it to hospital, but I barely dragged myself up to Sutton. It was good I had to belly drag myself to hospital otherwise I would maybe have died in the house as I had not eaten for close to 2 weeks or drank anything it was difficult swallowing or pushing anything through the mouth to the wounded areas.

That morning it had snowed heavily but I had to use the only energy that was left to get out and get into the train to go for the 6th last radiotherapy. I wanted to get through with it as it had taken its toll on me.

I made the mistake of entering a bus that was not passing by the hospital gate, as I was running late and thought to jump on this other bus I could arrive faster, I was mistaken. When the bus dropped me just to walk about 200 metres to the hospital it was like climbing Mount Kilimanjaro, in Tanzania. I had to rest several times but eventually arrived.

When my turn came to get on the driving seat on to the radiotherapy machine, I was all over the place. The radiographers were quite concerned that they told me to get down. They brought a wheelchair and wheeled into a consultation room to wait for the consultant to make decisions.

Eventually, the consultant came and immediately put me into admission. However, because there were no bed spaces in Sutton and much more I was a St George's University Hospital main patient, I was transferred to St Georges hospital. I was wheeled out of the hospital into the waiting ambulance to take me St George's University Hospital for admission.

At St George's University Hospital, I was taken to A&E for admission. They put cannula on me after quite a time and then had a blood test. They tried to insert a tube to begin feeding me via the tube however due to the wound inside by where the tube was to pass it was too painful. I had never seen such green bile coming out of a human-like it did on me that night. They tried to insert the tube through my nose 4 times, and they failed then I was wheeled to a wardroom for admission. I was then put on IV treatment that started to be around the clock 24/7.

The first night I was initially booked into a temporary ward as they waited for a bed in the cancer wing. I was put on IV treatment. My brother joined me there as he told me to let him know if I had left the A&E and which ward I had been put in. I tell you sometimes people are sceptical of the tracking technology. But on me, I can assure you that this monitoring between me and my brother was quite beneficial as he could know my location and would at split-second contact me to check if all is alright. This day he knew things were not fine as I had moved from one hospital to another and was still around the A&E till late. That night I was moved to the cancer ward where I spent the night. My brother escorted me to the ward and left me for the night.

20/03/2018: The second day they tried to take me for another tube insertion for feeding but it could not go in. I tried to tell them if they could feed me other ways, but they told me quite often it is the last resort, but it is not one of the safest to do. I was kept on 24 hours IV treatment and the introduced pain killer morphine that I could request anytime I felt pain.

21/03/2018: On the third day they again tried to insert a tube with a consultant present, but it did not work. They then abandoned the idea as I waited for the nutritionist to see how I was doing. On this day the 21/03/2018, they had to take me back for radiotherapy to finish up the course. I was taken by an ambulance to RMH and then back to St George's University Hospital once the treatment was done. I was still using the

Rowan machine.

22/03/2018: On 4th day I was again taken to the RMH for radiotherapy via the ambulance system and brought back. Each time I went was the only time they disconnected the IV treatment otherwise it was on full time the moment I was on my bed.

23/03/2018: On the fifth day the nutrition came to see me and then they opted not to go ahead with the tube as I had now some energy and because I was on morphine it could numb the pain a bit and I could eat some soft food and drink some little water however little but it was better than nothing. I still went for the radiotherapy for my sessions.

24/03/2018: On the sixth day I went for the radiotherapy and then came back and things were a bit looking positive as I could get up off the bed and try a few tricks or two of venturing into the toilets and back. This was now my 25th-26/03/2018 was a weekend so there was no movement for radiotherapy but stayed in the hospital with 24/7 IV treatment

27/03/2018: was my second last radiotherapy and went to RMH and came back to St George's University Hospital.

28/03/2018: was my last day of radiotherapy and qualified for the 30 sessions. That day I was taken by ambulance and then wheeled in the radiotherapy room. After that, I came out, signed off. Then as I was being wheeled in a wheelchair to go to the ambulance, just as we were about to enter the lift, there was this old lady walking with two sticks. We entered the lift together. Within this split second, she told us she was 91 years and she had just been declared cancer-free. It was amazing. We congratulated her. But you could imagine I was being wheeled and she was on her two feet walking. Such is the amazing things that left an impact on me that with this thing 'Cee' not all is lost whatever the age, there is always hope, faith. It is about believing that all would be fine.

29/03/2018: the medical professions felt I was strong enough to be discharged. I was now discharged back to the GP and referred to the District nurses for community assessment.

xxxv. **The '*Mythical Journey*' of Hospitalisation.**

On the 19th March 2018, I had to be admitted in hospital as a result of dehydration, no eating and heavy loss of weight. By the time I was admitted I had lost 13 kilograms of body weight. That morning I went normally for my daily radiotherapy. I could hardly make it to hospital, but I barely dragged myself up to Sutton. It was good I had to belly drag myself to hospital otherwise I would maybe have died in the house as I had not eaten drunk anything for close to 2 weeks. It was difficult swallowing or pushing anything through the mouth to the wounded areas.

That morning it had snowed heavily but I had to use the only energy that was left to get out and get into the train to go for the 6th and last radiotherapy. I wanted to get over with it as it had taken its toll on me.

I made the mistake of entering a bus that was not passing by the hospital gate, as I was running late and thought to jump on this other bus I could arrive faster. I was mistaken. When the bus dropped me just to walk about 200 metres to the hospital was like climbing Mt Kilimanjaro, in Tanzania. I had to rest several times but eventually arrived.

When my turn came to get on the driving seat of the radiotherapy machine, I was all over the place. The radiographers were so gravely concerned that they told me to get down. A radiographer brought a wheelchair and I was wheeled into a consultation room to wait for the consultant to make decisions.

Eventually, the consultant came and immediately put me into admission. However, because there were no bed spaces in Sutton I was transferred to St Georges Hospital. I was wheeled out of the hospital into the waiting ambulance to take me St George's University Hospital for admission.

At St George's University Hospital, I was taken to A&E for admission. They put cannula on me after quite a time and then had a blood test. They tried to insert a tube to begin feeding me via the tube. However, due to the wound inside where the tube was meant to pass it was too painful. I had never seen such green bile coming out of a human being like it did on me that night. They tried and failed to insert the tube through my nose 4 times. Then I was wheeled to a wardroom for admission. I was then put on IV treatment that started to be around the clock 24/7.

The first night I was initially booked into a temporary ward as they waited for a bed in the cancer wing. I was put on IV treatment. My brother joined me there as he told me to let him know if I had left the A&E and which ward I had been put in. I tell you sometimes people are sceptical of the tracking technology. But I can assure them that this monitoring between me and my brother was quite beneficial as he could know my location and would at split-second contact me to check if all was alright. This day he knew things were not fine as I had moved from one hospital to another and was still around the A&E till late. That night I was moved to the cancer ward where I spent the night. My brother escorted me to the ward and left me for the night.

20/03/2018: The second day the clinicians tried to take me for another tube insertion for feeding, but it could not go in. I tried to tell them if they could feed me other ways, but they told me quite often it is the last resort, but it was not one of the safest to do. I was kept on 24 hours IV treatment and also the introduced pain killer morphine that I could request anytime I felt pain.

21/03/2018: On the third day the clinicians again tried to insert a tube with a consultant present, but it did not work. They then abandoned the idea as I waited for the nutritionist to see how I was doing. On this day the 21/08/2018, they had to take me back for radiotherapy to finish the course. I was taken by an ambulance to RMH and then back to St George's University Hospital once the treatment was done. I was still using the Rowan machine.

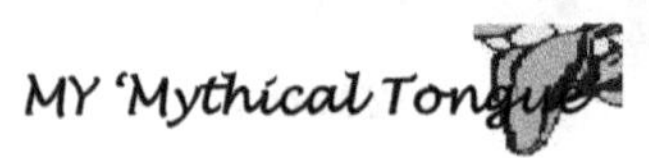

22/03/2018: On 3rd day I was again taken to the RMH for radiotherapy via the ambulance system and brought back. Each time I went was the only time they disconnected the IV treatment otherwise it was on full time the moment I was on my bed.

23/03/2019: On the 4th day the nutritionist came to see me and opted not to go ahead with the tube as I had now some energy and because I was on morphine it could numb the pain a bit and I could eat some soft food and drink some little water however little. It was better than nothing. I still went for the radiotherapy for my sessions.

24/03/2019: On the 5th day I went for the radiotherapy and then came back and things were a bit looking positive as I could get up off the bed and try a few tricks or two of venturing into the toilets and back. This was now my 25th-

26/03/2019: Was a weekend so there was no movement for radiotherapy, but I stayed in the hospital with 24/7 IV treatment

27/03/2019: Was my 2nd last radiotherapy and went to RMH and came back to St George's University Hospital.

28/03/2019: Was my last day of radiotherapy and qualified for the 30sessions. That day I was taken by ambulance and then wheeled in the radiotherapy room. After that, I came out, signed off. Then as I was being wheeled in a wheelchair to go to the ambulance, just as we were about to enter the lift, this old lady was walking with two sticks. We entered the lift together. Within this split second, she told us she was 91 years and she had just been declared cancer-free. It was amazing. We congratulated her. But you could imagine I was being wheeled and she was on her two feet walking. Such is the amazing things that left an impact on me that with this thing 'C' not all is lost whatever the age, there is always hope, faith. It is about believing that all would be fine.

29/03/2019: The medical professions felt I was strong enough to be discharged. I was now discharged back to the GP and referred to the District nurses for community assessment.

xxxvi. **14/04/2018 Reflection as I was doing some *'Mythical write-up'*.**

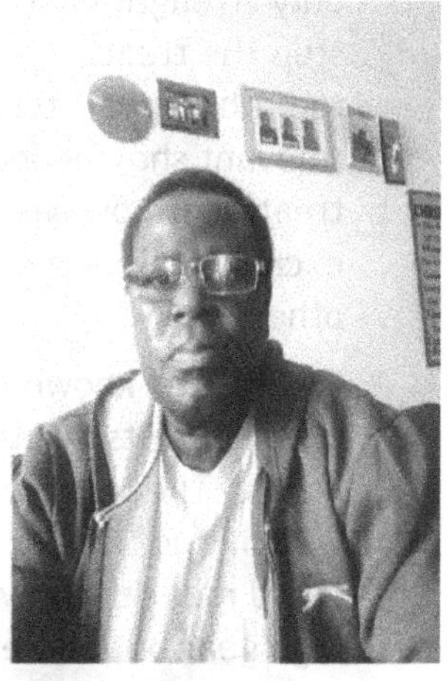

xxxvii. **A *'mythical interaction'* with my *'Mythical Ki Moyimo'*... the 'Cee' patient,**

It is that once in a lifetime that when you feel you are down and out, but you know someone else needs your strength to get out of the deep hole. Such was the time when *'mythical Ki Moyimo'* made contact with me that she was undergoing similar problems of that thing 'Cee'.

On understanding that she was also undergoing the same, I cried, on her disclosure that her daughter a few months before that she had also passed away following a lengthy battle with 'Cee'. I was so devastated, but I said fine; I looked helpless but what could I do in my helpless situations to make someone else's situation look different. I had also lost my son a year before I would assume, I knew how she felt having that lose and currently being in this predicament.

I had to get up wipe off my tears and get up and stand up to hold her like a war-torn hero. The only thing I could do was to encourage her to hold on to that hope however little, however hopeless the situation looked. She told me she was having a rough time as the treatment was taking its toll. I shared with her my coping mechanism; my difficulty was eating but what I could force down my throat to stay alive. She was not sure what was going on, but I offered her the only strength I had left to cry on. I told her she should not stop the treatment as she was undergoing both chemo and radiotherapy. I told her based on my experience that it was relevant she needed to pick herself up and continue the treatment however painful and energy less she felt. We were exchanging our dilemmas via WhatsApp and assuring each other.

I had never known that when you are faced with similar predicaments whatever it is you close ranks and support each other. The last time I felt this way was when I wanted to lose weight and used to walk and run all over London roads. You could meet those who were at the beginning and some now in high gear but all helping each other. This is the way I felt along the way when I came face to face with those faced with 'Cee' issues. They tend all to learn and help one another. It is another family in itself.

Below I have to share a few exchanges I had with Ki Moyimo in order to lend support.

"[19:48, 16/5/2018] Ki Moyimo ...: Hi Jesse, hp u ar ok. We were meant to talk but this& that kept coming up. Munange I was left with 8 sessions of radio having finished 17. Then I had a setback yesterday.

[19:49, 16/5/2018] Ki Moyimo ...: Yes, I am in a storied building where the network is v poor. Let me just text do not worry.

[19:50, 16/5/2018] ofano759: Sorry to hear that.

[19:51, 16/5/2018] Ki Moyimo ...: I was hospitalised yesterday coz I got severe vascular imbalance/motion. Radio inflamed my ears and now I can't walk or turn quick this way or that way.

[19:51, 16/5/2018] ofano759: Radiotherapy is very radical it drains especially when coming to the end of treatment.

[19:51, 16/5/2018] Ki Moyimo ...: I feel everything moving

around me and prefer to sit than lie down.

[19:53, 16/5/2018] ofano759: you need to have surgical socks in your legs 24/7 to avoid clot

[19:53, 16/5/2018] Ki Moyimo ...: I believe u. Coz the way am feeling its terrible. I remembered u and said this is it.

[19:53, 16/5/2018] ofano759: are you eating and drinking at all.

[19:54, 16/5/2018] ofano759: so those side effects are normal it is just about managing it to finalise your treatment.

[19:54, 16/5/2018] Ki Moyimo ...: Those I don't have. My late daughter had but they are small/too tight.

[19:55, 16/5/2018] Ki Moyimo ...: Now I am, but yet I was over vomiting

[19:56, 16/5/2018] ofano759: you need to buy medium or large size. they do measurements and get right size

[19:56, 16/5/2018] Ki Moyimo ...: But I didn't do radiotherapy yesterday & today. I have no energy I tell u.

[19:58, 16/5/2018] ofano759: when I had my relapse, I stopped for two days but they took me back once they had stabilised me.

[19:59, 16/5/2018] Ki Moyimo ...: I wonder if that can be done here. She used to get them from outside.

[20:00, 16/5/2018] ofano759: You will get over it once the just stabilised you and finish it. slowly you will pick up again, but it is draining.

[20:00, 16/5/2018] Ki Moyimo ...: Oh ok. I might have to do that then.

[20:00, 16/5/2018] ofano759: They come ready-made they just measure and give you the right size.

[20:01, 16/5/2018] Ki Moyimo ...: Ok. I get it.

[20:03, 16/5/2018] ofano759: yah because with the treatment they require it to be consistent, so you need to get back to it once stable a bit as the feelings is part of the

treatment and it is just side effects but not sickness.

[20:05, 16/5/2018] ofano759: I am now much better. I will be going to my sister's in Sweden for some few weeks then come back for normal review they will be coming to Uganda in June before I come back for final tests and result.

[20:05, 16/5/2018] ofano759: You may need food nutrients to help you pick up energy level

[20:06, 16/5/2018] Ki Moyimo ...: Like what?

[20:07, 16/5/2018] Ki Moyimo ...: Oh, that will be very good for u for sure. U need the rest.

[20:10, 16/5/2018] ofano759: you need to check with good chemist who may stock or get a nutritionist to support you with what is good. But ordinary one is obuseera, soya porridge, passion fruits juice, molokony soup.

[20:11, 16/5/2018] Ki Moyimo ...: Oh ok. Those I have been eating.

[20:12, 16/5/2018] ofano759: then you are on right path

[20:15, 16/5/2018] Ki Moyimo ...: That's how things are moving my dear

[20:16, 16/5/2018] Ki Moyimo ...: But I pray and know that I will be fine.

[20:17, 16/5/2018] ofano759: you will be fine just finish up the course of treatment; all will be well we trust in God bless

[20:17, 16/5/2018] Ki Moyimo ...: Amen and thanks

[20:18, 16/5/2018] ofano759: good night

[05:35, 17/5/2018] Ki Moyimo ...: Good morning. Hp u slept well? I have improved & still grateful for the info u gave me yesy.

[05:36, 17/5/2018] Ki Moyimo ...: Yesterday...

[05:46, 17/5/2018] Ki Moyimo ...: Am just worried about the bills here I would ask u to assist me a bit, but u must be in the same boat, I guess. I stopped working long time back so

lacking funds for this and that esp. for medication as u know here. U think u can help however little?

[20:47, 25/5/2018] Ki Moyimo ...: Hi there. I am better though still having dizziness & lack of appetite. I resumed radiotherapy after missing out 5 days. Now am remaining with 4 sessions. I hp I will feel better after completion. It's not a joke for sure.

[21:09, 25/5/2018] ofano759: Sorry about that you will overcome

[21:11, 25/5/2018] ofano759: If you can eat anything do. Me up to now still weak but improving. I am in Sweden."

xxxviii. A '*Mythical Journey*' of Round two of disclosure

I had not disclosed to my '*mythical sister Swallah*' from Sweden about my ailment. There was a day when I was going to RMH for my radiotherapy, she then sent me a message asking for my son's contact number. I froze as I thought the 'cat' had been let out of the bag and she was trying to look for information and/or to confirm. I gave her the contact and at the same time, because I was on the train, I sent the pictures to show her I was up and about.

Anyway, I realised later that it was not the case. So eventually when I learnt she was coming to London for a week's course I had to disclose to her. She did not take it lightly. But I kept on reassuring her that I had finished treatment and I was out of the hospital. And all was well. She then told me when she comes, we shall go back with her to Sweden. I could not say no as I knew how much she cares about and for me. There was time again I was not well in 2005 when I finished being hospitalised and was at home she had wanted me to have gone to Sweden to recuperates but I declined because by then the children were young and they required me to be around whenever going and coming back from school. This time I had no excuse, so I had to book myself in to go back with her to Sweden. She decided to come with my in-law so that they would support me to go back together.

xxxix. My first '*mythical get-together*' at the '*mythical Pe'Op*' Ambassadors' house.

That day my brother picked me up however before that he kept on checking if I was strong enough to go out to the '*mythical ambassador's house*' as the wife had lost a father and had come back and we needed to get together. That day when I went there my '*mythical Ambassador Pe'OP*', welcomed us and asked me that I looked well and was asking me about this 'thing' people a scared to call by name hence he is the one who brought for me the letter 'Cee' '*mythical word*'. I told him that I am like this because of him. He had taught me how to fight positive fights without being relentless. I stayed there for over two hours and enjoyed the company, and this was my first step out to the recovery process.

I met my '*mythical Hon. Acuti Lwani*' who had also undergone major medical issues and had come out of the other side of the tunnel, that was one of the my defining hopes in determination to came to the other side once the medical professions had made the assurance they could contain the illness but it was about me getting the determination to pull through. So, I looked and held on the two to get me through. Sometimes when going through some of these situations you look for any sort of alignment, any sort of something to cling to that hope and faith. And these two offered me those '*mythical hopes*' and faith to believe in the medical professions.

xl. The '*Mythical Journey of Recovery*' - Journey to Sweden.

On the morning of the Swedish journey. I was picked from my house by my sister and brother-in-law for flight via Stansted to Sweden. After we had checked in, we then had a few chats generally about things. It came a time when my '*mythical Swallah sister*' had to confront me with some issues about my health and bereavement and other issues. When I had to open to them about the issues I had faced, my *'mythical brother-in-law GOOK'*, did a runner into the toilets. My *'mythical Swallah sister'* told me that often he does not want to go into details of such things as he is so fragile. I then told my *'mythical Swallah sister'* that, I do not want to be sitting there having a conversation with her and when my brother-in-law appears then it would look like we were either discussing him or gossiping about something he should not be privy to.

However, I realised that my *'mythical brother-in-law'* broke down, in tears and went away. So, we left the discussion for another day. We boarded the aircraft and left for Sweden. Throughout the flight, they kept checking on my welfare. As this was my first flight since undergoing treatment, they were a bit apprehensive. However, there were no issues and we landed safety.

We then passed by one of a *'mythical family friend'* Dr Oku, who picked us up at the airport, thereafter we moved to their home in Orebro.

I felt loved and my *'mythical Swallah sister'* at all times tried her best to look after me though I told her there was only so much I could eat; however, she still used her maternal instinct to force food on me. In fact, after my three weeks stay, I had gained three extra kilos from 78 kilos to 81 kilos. I thanked her for being a good mum to me for the duration.

During my stay, I had to confront my *'mythical brother-in-law mythical GOOK'* about him not wanting to listen to some of the issues I needed to air out. Often when he came back from work, we could sit in the lounge up to late and we talked, and I talked, and he listened for the first three days he broke down. He cried for each of the three days. After that, I saw him now feeling better in himself. I knew there were certain things he never wanted to hear, listen to but I told him if I cannot offload some of those things to him then who else should I do it too. I have trusted him for donkey years including giving him, my *'mythical Swallah sister'*. That is the level of trust.

This made me realise that often if you see people putting up a front, sometimes, in essence, they are trying create a screen to avoid being confronted with what is unpalatable or sometimes not wanting to hurt the unknown feelings a person has had to deal with or not wanting to expose.

We then made a trip to Stockholm for a weekend away with him and met other Ugandan those were quite therapeutic time and helped me to feel that recovery was being delivered.

During my stay, our '*mythical family friend*' Dr Oku passed by as he had come to see me and talk about how I was feeling following the treatments. I asked him about some of the things I experienced during the treatment and he told me that sometimes chemotherapy ends up treating other alignments you have though it cannot be given for such alignment. Because it was funny that part of the side effects was that I was meant to lose hair but instead I grow afro hair. During my stay in the hospital, my pressure drugs were also discontinued as my pressure was stable. He explained that during treatment the blood vessels can be enlarged or thinned so there was the most likely scenario that my veins may have enlarged during the course of treatment.

During the time I was with my '*mythical Swallah sister*'. She then discussed with me that; it was the best time to disclose to our '*mythical commander sister*' about my illness. I had wanted to hold on until I was in Uganda but she told me I needed to disclose to her because at least now I had finished treatment and has even travelled.

At this point, we agreed, and we rang her talked and disclosed to her. We are aware of how she would normally act when she receives such information. We, therefore, knew it could have happened the same way hence, we disclosed to her and reassured her that all was okay, though she was not fully convinced. So, day-in-day-out she kept on sending messages to our '*mythical Swallah sister*' asking how I woke up, how I am during the day, how I am in the evening, whether I have had anything to eat, if so what quantity. My '*mythical sister*' called Commander was now on overdrive in a per second, per second telephone calls to my '*mythical Swallah sister*' who had to give her the updates. That is the level of how our *'mythical sister'* called Commander acts in any such scenarios.

Swallah and me in Sweden Stockholm

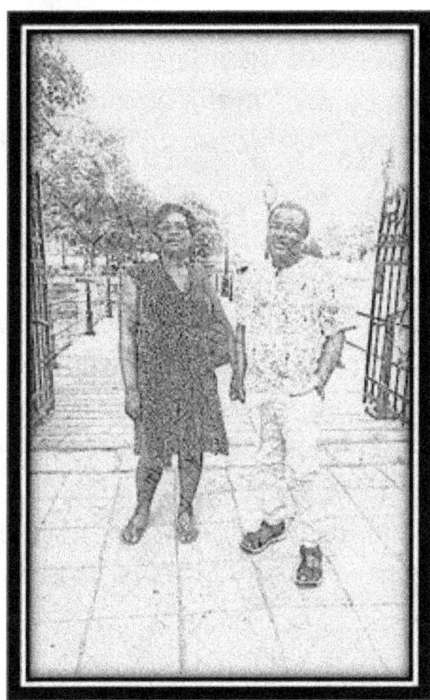

26/05/2018 – With Owuya

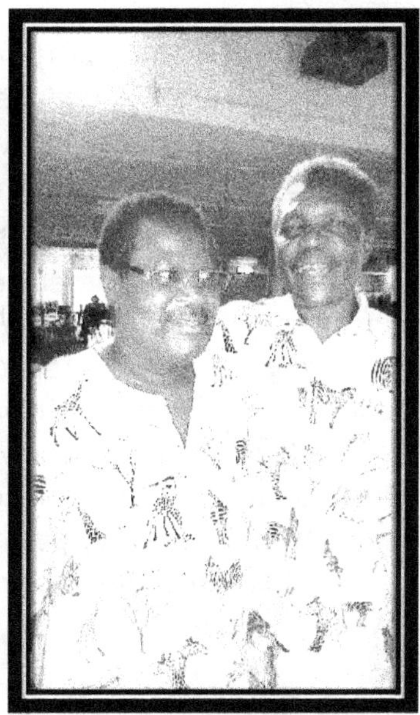

Sweden Stockholm.

xli. *'Mythical Journey back'* to the UK from Sweden.

The journey back to the UK was more to do with going for review and then getting off to Uganda as now at least there was the aspect that I could travel having made the trial run. In fact, going to Sweden and also to Uganda was the brainchild of my Swedes parents who felt I needed to make the trips after all my *'mythical brother-in-law'* would be in Uganda and would help me to recover and a company in return. So, on the day I came back from Sweden to the UK was the day my *'mythical brother-in-law'* also was taking off to go to Uganda.

After seeing the consultant on the 15th of June 2018 and happy with my recovery we agreed for the next appointment to be in three months, hence the need to take a break and recover from this whole process. So, Uganda here I came, battered, fragile, weak, lost but still strong at heart and ready to confront the new world.

xlii. *'Mythical Journey to Uganda'*

On the 16th of June 2018, I took off to Uganda arriving on the 17th of June 2018 and picked up by my *'mythical cousin Dr Otek'*. The same day I arrived my *'mythical cousin Dr Otek'* left that night for Canada.

So, on Monday the 18th of June 2018 I visited my *'mythical sister-in-law'* and thereafter had made an appointment to meet up with my *'mythical sister called commander'* at the Lugogo ground, but after some time I realised she was not coming. However, my *'mythical commander'* did not appear. I can only suspect that knowing her she did not want to face me head-on unless she had made a consultation with someone else and interrogated that person, she cannot stand the first-hand sight. I am sure she was not a privy to any other person as I was in Uganda.

xliii. Disclosure to *'mythical brother Jenk'*

I met up with my *'mythical brother Jenk'*. We had lunch together and I had to disclose to him as to what I have undergone for the last one year. I reassured him that though I have come back with no results it was reassuring from the medical point of view.

The next day we left Kampala City very early with my *'mythical nephew'* he escorted me up to Tororo Town and then to Lwala P'Obona village, of which I met my *'mythical mother'* for the fast time since I left her a year back after burying my son. What a year of a roller coaster. However, my mother was not aware of my illness, so we hugged as usually welcoming me home.

My niece was also home the one who held the fort during the

trying times. That was my *'mythical Sipi Choices'*.

My uncle the *'mythical Amunoni'* then came around to drop for me the car I could use while around.

xliv. Disclosure to *'mythical sister Nyari Ochido Milyong'*

On Friday the 22nd June 2018, drove to town met up with my *'mythical brother-in-law Gook'* who was around to offer me necessary support. I picked my *'mythical sister Nyari Ochido Milyong'*. As I drove back with her, I felt it was much better to talk to her in the car while driving the two of us. Just as we were slowing from Misukiire hill, into the swamp and bridge demarcating Misukiire village and into Kidera village I pulled the bomb out of my *'mythical tongue'* and crushed it into her. I felt a vacuum-like environment in the car as if something had just evaporated. I believe if heaven could open for her, it would have done at that critical moment. However, I reassured her that all was being taken care of, as I had just come back home to change the environment and recover. I do not know what or how she felt when I threw the bomb at her in an enclosed environment that she could not run out, she could not wail, she could not hit me that what she was hearing was not true. I assumed in her mind she was thinking maybe she should have jumped on her usual *'Bodaboda'* to reach home than be listening to the bombarding words that came from my *'mythical tongue'*.

I then checked with her if I could disclose it to mother. She at that point, and; point-blank refused and said just enjoy your time with her. I accepted as this was coming from the very top hierarchy of the *'Mythical* tongue' of my *'mythical Nyari Ochido Milyong'*, and left things at that. I am very much aware of her protecting mother. She is the main career and she would not want such bombs to be landing at the doorsteps and she has no way of controlling.

I pitted her as now she was going to have two fragile people in the same household, and she had to pull up all her stops in order to support both. But anyway, such is the nature of

'Mythical Nyari Ochido', they will never falter in what they are doing as they are very passionate and caring to the level they forget their own illnesses and issues affecting them. Thumbs up *'Mythical Nyari Ochido Milyong'*, for they say caregivers go through a lot than what you see and or tell you. They often try to hold the fort even when there are punches and dripping. They hold it for sanity to prevail.

xlv. Disclosure to my *'mythical Waya Mangulata'*

On Saturday the 08/07/2018, When my *'mythical Waya Mangulata'* came to see me, she was not yet aware of my situation. She found me in the bedroom when she arrived. I went out and exchanged greetings with her. To my understanding after exchanging greeting and left she was not happy with what she saw. I understand she asked my *'mythical sister Nyari Ochido Milyong'* whether I was actually fine. *Nyari Ochido Milyong*, so I understand told her to have said: *'...well let him tell you himself...'*

I called my *'mythical Waya Mangulata'* to come to the bedroom and we had a chat. I was in bed and she knelt by my bedside at the foot. I disclosed to my *'mythical Waya Mangulata'*. When we were talking, she burst in tears and prayed that I should get better. I reassured her that all will be well as I have already undergone treatment and currently, I am recovering and recuperating. She then disclosed to me something else about one of her own who underwent a similar situation and treatment that lasted close to 4 years. At that point, she pulled out 20,000 Ugsh - and gave to me to wish me well. I was so touched and grateful and a tear or two got squeezed past my eyes. Often it is difficult to believe as people assume that its, we in the diaspora who hold money to give and not to receive this was so touching.

A year later when I went back to Uganda in October 2019, following two years after diagnosis I happened to have again interacted with my *'mythical Waya Mangulata'* who informed me following serious chat about my health that; when she

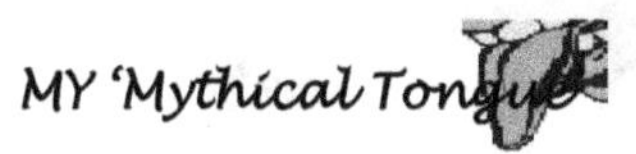

came to visit me that time my *'mythical mother'* confided in her and told her the person she had come to see does not look well. However, she kept a brave face as my *'mythical mother'* told her to let her see me and then let her know. So, during our conversation then and now she told me when she went back to her. She was asked what was wrong with me, but she declined to disclose our discussion, she said all was well.

xlvi. My Mythical Disclosure to My *'Mythical Daughter Ka-Landlady'*

I did not get the courage to disclosure to my *'mythical daughter Ka-landlady'*, directly however I disclosed via a third party who told her and from my understanding, she was dejected, she felt he was going to lose a father she has hardly known. She kept away from me. It was only at the intervention of My *'Mythical BNO'* is when on my last night in Uganda she came and we had a brief chat. However, upon my second return, she was in a position to come and stayed with me at Lwala P'Obona and we blended well. At this point is when she felt the dad could live and still alive. We had good bonding time and felt grateful that she could come around and had daughter-dad moments. For the first time, we had Xmas together with my *'mythical grandson' 'Mythical Jojo'*. We had our moments that was best of both worlds.

xlvii. The *'mythical building'* of my son's grave a year on.

Part of going back to Uganda was also to finish building my son's grave as it was more than a year ago after burying him we had to leave back for the UK so it was not fully done. So I embarked on sorting out his headstone with my *'mythical nephew Ofedi'* It was also a therapeutic process for me for recovery. I felt I needed to finish the unfinished business as I believed if I go today and will not have done his grave, I would not guarantee someone else would do it sorting my son's grave. After sorting his grave, it also coincided with his and my mum's birthday, so we had to combine all the ceremonies and we celebrated it. Also, in a sense, I was celebrating situations I had gone through and still around to witness this day. So, we called the priest and had prayers on the 14th July 2018, we combined the two birthdays and commemorating the Late.

My *'Mythical sister'* called Commander came around and we spent a week with her for the duration. As you are aware of my *'mythical sister'* called Commander, she was asking questions, I showed her my medical records on the Phone App and she was sort of not convinced. She kept probing as if there were things, I was still hiding from her.

xlviii. *'Mythical events'.*

One time I was joking with my mother about her not eating and after I had left she confronted my *'mythical sister Nyari Ochido'* that her visitor was telling her she is not eating but she should also see that I was not eating.

I fell sick twice while in Uganda. The first once I had very serious diarrhoea that I had never experienced like that in my life. Literary there was no stopping. Eventually, *'mythical Nyari Ochido Milyong'* brought me some tablets from town.

The second time I fell sick I could hardly breathe or walk. I tried to hold it but eventually, I had to give in and told *'mythical Sipi Choices'* to explore options of taking me to town for medical treatment as my right upper rib cage. When I arrived in town, I found a lot of medical professionals including my *'mythical Waya Anyane'* and my *'mythical 'nephew Roberto'* waiting for me. I was told to get a scan but even before then they diagnosed the illness and gave me the medication to buy. We then went to town for a scan. The scan proved there was an infection and it corresponded with what medication I was told to buy and take. My *'Mythical Waya Anyane'* was walking like she was stepping on hot charcoal directing things as if I was near to passing away. I couldn't believe when doors were being opened things were being done at the whim and medications being bought without being asked for money. Such is the time when you know that people care about saving lives and not caring how they do it.

xlix. Visiting my *'Mythical uncle ASO'*

While still in Uganda I went to Maruki in Paya to visit my *'mythical maternal uncle'' Mythical ASO'.* He was not well and was bed-bound. I went around as I knew he had undergone similar situations like mine, and he was now bed-bound. I went there and disclosed to him my own illness in order to support him hold on to hope and faith in the treatment. I shared with him some tips or two how to deal with his situations. He was very gratefully for the disclosure.

l. My *'mythical journey'* back to the UK

I arrived back into the UK on the 3rd of August 2018 and met up with my brother formerly known as Seven-Thirty, who picked me at the airport and drove me home.

li. Meeting the consultant.

On the 10/08/2018 I met up with the consultant to see how I was doing and to book in for the Pet-scan to get the final result following the treatment.

lii. The Introduction and wedding of my mythical niece Miss-N 'the incoming *'Mythical Commander'* on the 25/08/2018 and the 28th/08/2018

In the process of waiting for the scan, we had an introduction and wedding ceremony of my *'mythical niece Miss-N'*. It was an enjoyable moment. Our families in and out of UK congregated and enjoyed each other's company. We had good times, good laughs and the company on both occasions were electric.

I met my *'mythical Brother Kitakwano Ongeri Oruko Sokosi'*, during the ceremonies, which both of us were charged to conduct. I had to disclose too to him about my illness in the last year. We almost exchanged blows. He was not amused. He asked me why I did not keep him in the loop. But I told him I had to manage the information. In the end, he felt fine and told him I will be getting my results in due course and will update him

Many of my relatives were around and gave me hope that a year on all would be well. We danced two nights away on each occasion.

liii. Attending PET-Scan III

On the 29th August 2018, I attended the pet scan I had the normal rituals as the previous two scans.

liv. *'Mythical result'* of PET-scan and treatment.

On the 07/09/2018 I went for my appointment for the result for the final say on the position of 'Cee'. The appointment was for 10.00 am. When I entered the room, my Consultant was beaming and gave me the most positive result after a year of agony. He said the scan has shown complete response to the disease and there was no evidence of metabolic activity. In a second I walked out of the room I am not sure whether I run, walked, crawled or did what. However, what I remember I sat down on the bench by the entrance of the hospital. As was pondering what to do. They say telepathy speaks, indeed this one came working truthfully as my *'mythical Swallah sister'* called me. I wondered what the telepathy in the call was. I avoided disclosing to her the result. So, I told her I would call her in one hour. By then I was moving to my *'mythical brother's''* - formerly called Seven-Thirty, home in east London. When I got out of the train, I then rang my *'mythical Swallah sister'* and we chatted but did not disclose anything yet.

While at my *'mythical brother's place'*, that is when once I disclosed to my brother and sister in law. Then my brother called my *Swallah sister* to tell her I was around, and I wanted to talk to her. That is when I disclosed to her the result and she was over the moon. We then called my *'Waya Mangulata'* and also put her in the know as she was very worried about me.

lv. Our *'Mythical Journey'* together with my long-time *'mythical friend'* Ed'Kan

'Mythical Ed'Kan' has been my long-time friend. We met at Caltec Academy Makerere while pursuing out 'A' levels in Uganda. We also happened to have lived in the village of Bugolobi, the outskirts of Kampala metropolitan. We have had a lot in common. We used to have our own silly moments and support each other in our own *'mythical stupid way'*. When I moved to the UK we stayed in touch. He moved with his family for a two-year work-related before going back to Uganda. He became the Godfather of my last-born son, Kaio X R '01. While I was undergoing my treatment and recovery, somehow, he also had his own fight with the 'Cee'. I had not known he has always kept me by his side this deep. Hence, when he was diagnosed with Cancer and undergoing pain, he wrote to me the message below very touching.

> *"Hi, Jesse. For the last few months, I kept something from you because I wanted not to worry you but if things had gone wrong you would still get a message from me. Keep to yourself and*

Agnes till I come out openly. I spent the last two weeks in AgaKhan Hospital, Nairobi City, after a successful operation to remove my prostate as I was in the early stages of cancer. Stayed long because of many other complications. Now at my sisters in Nairobi. Thanks be to GOD. Please check your PSA levels to know how you stand. If you don't check please do. This I say because I love you my brother. Have a nice day".

WhatsApp on the 26/10/2018.

End of message.

I had to get on to him. I rang him and found him in pain having just been operated, but he kept the faith and we reassured each other that I had also undergone cancer treatment and recovering. I had felt while in Uganda, we could have met but it did not happen as we kept on missing each other. Sometimes when one searches for true friendship is not about the good a person offers but the shoulder to cry on. We are both now classified as survivors of that whatever period God allows to continue being survivors we shall survive as bet mates.

lvi. A *'Mythical Testimony'* presentation at the Holy Redeemer Church on Sunday the 04/11/2018

I had wanted to do this presentation in only one minute, but Ian told me I should not speak very fast, so I took note.

My name is JESSE ALECHO.

I can be Identified as the father of The Late IOA father, and/or AOA's dad.

I am grateful to Ian to allow me to stand in front of you to give my gratitude and testimony to the congregation of the Holy Redeemer Church.

I was not expecting that a year to date, I would be standing here.

For over a year now you have been praying for The Alecho's family after IOA's death,

You have been praying for AOA due to what he has gone through.

And you have been praying for me due to what I have been undergoing.

In September of last year, I acquired another name.

I became A CANCER PATIENT.

I was diagnosed with Esophageal Cancer.

I have never been so grateful and thankful to God that has enabled me to stand in front of you, the congregation of The Holy Redeemer Church and to narrate this to you.

In Matthew Chapter 7 verse.7-10

[7] "Ask, and it will be given to you; seek, and you will find; knock, and it will be opened to you.

[8] For everyone who asks receives, and he who seeks finds, and to him who knocks it will be opened.

[9] Or what man is there among you who, if his son asks for bread, will give him a stone?

[10] Or if he asks for a fish, will he give him a serpent?

You prayed for my treatment to go well.

You prayed for my recovery.

You prayed day in and day out for me, my immediate and wider family.

[11] By holding on to faith, hope and you holding me, in your prayers: -

I went through SIX MONTHS of Intensive Treatment that involved: -

- 5 SESSIONS OF CHEMOTHERAPY.
- 30 SESSIONS OF RADIOTHERAPY.

[12] And Hospitalisation for two weeks: -

- When I could not WALK,

- When I could not EAT OR DRINK anything.
- I managed to come out of it all.
- On the 7th of September 2018, I was declared CANCER-FREE.
- All due to your thoughts, prayers to support my faith in God our Lord and hope in the medical field to bring me back to life.
- I close by reading Psalm 27 Verse 13

[13] I remain confident of this:

- I will see the goodness of the Lord
- in the land of the living.

With this, I would advise the Church Congregation and all those you happen to meet: - Please ask yourself and them: -

- How many times have you avoided knocking at your doctor's door, when you should have?
- How many times in the last 2 years have you accessed any medical help?

When faced with cancer or any other devastating illness.

> *"The best thing to do is take one day at a time, be positive, pick your head up when you are down and remember what may seem like the most devastating news in your life, can always open doors to a whole new world".*

HERE I AM your testimony.

04/11/2018: A very close friend of mine sent me this message on WhatsApp on the 26/10/2018.

And I read: -

"Hi Jesse. ……… [See Mythical **Our *'Mythical Journey'* together with my long-time *'mythical friend'* Ed'Kan]**

End of message

Please free to approach me and talk about anything you would like to know, that is why I am here because my other name is, A Cancer Survivor.

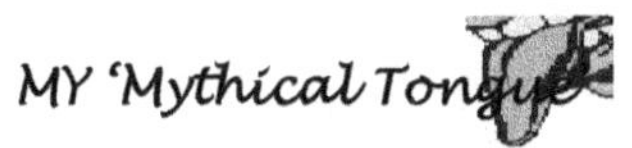

TOGETHER WE CAN BEAT CANCER.

Thank you, God bless, you all.

lvi My *'Mythical Journey'* back to Uganda

I had wanted to have gone back to Uganda immediately after the result but was persuaded by my *'mythical Swallah sister'* to go back with her in December so that they could be supportive as they would also be going back. She had proposed that I go back to Sweden to recuperate again before that but due to the expenses, I decided to wait and instead make the trip back to Uganda. So, we agreed and said we would meet in Uganda on the day of the flight landing.

During the time I was with my *'mythical niece Enid'* after I had rested, I had told her I would need a bit of Uganda Waragi. However, during our chat that is when she asked me how come, I had come to Uganda so frequently a few months after the other. I had now to explain to her the circumstances of my illness and my need to recuperate. Alas, Hell broke loose! Japadhola says *'Apee!!'* meaning *'Oh My!!'* I had forgotten that my *'mythical tongue'* twisted and spat out the wrong words in the eyes of the: I had not known to be another *'mythical Commander'*. I tried to put the *'mythical Uganda waragi'* request back, but it was all over the floor, running riot. For years I had not had a chance of having a commander by my side. I met another one that day, I curled in my baby-self. She was taking no, no sense. She told me her being of the professionals in the medical field she is not going to allow me to take that *'mythical Uganda Waragi'* or any *'mythical alcohol'* for that matter. And for that, she closed that door of any discussion of having any *'mythical alcoholic thing'* call it whatever name. I cowed into my *'mythical corner'* like a newborn *'mythical baby'* and accepted the Jopadhola saying that; *'Nyathi goyo buli... jadwong bende mielo'* (Meaning that a child can also drum, and an adult can also dance). It is not always one-way traffic. I realised that I had crossed the other side of the Rubicon now being told off and in the strongest term and unable to *'mythically cross back'*. It is the time I accepted to present day now to leave the dance hall for others, to also play their part.

We had also to fulfil a pledge as we had not seen our niece *'Mythical Enid'* since the age of 1. So, it would be good to pay her a visit in Entebbe Town before going back to Tororo.

So, on the 31/11/2018, my *'mythical Swallah sister'* was supposed to have landed the night before and me to land in the morning. I would have found her at our niece's place, then I would be picked up too and have lunch before proceeding to Kampala City. However, it was meant not to be as she missed her connections in Brussels. So instead I arrived first thing in the morning and she came in at night. So, by the time she arrived I had my jetlag done off with.

lvii Disclosure to my *'mythical Enid'*

Meeting my *'mythical Enid'* for the first time after donkey years since 1977 was not an easy task. The last time I saw her was when she still had milk teeth. When I first communicated to her on the phone it was like we had been meeting all along. That was the day I went to 125 Second Avenue to remit by a health care certificate.

It was as if living in *'mythical Switzerland'* and I was Me living in the *'Mythical United Kingdom'* had never drawn us apart. I felt at ease with her when we actually met when I arrived in the morning. She offered me shelter, I had a bath, nice good Uganda breakfast menu a brief chat and she allowed me to sleep off my jetlag.

When I woke up, she came around and to calm up my hopelessness *'mythical nerves'* I needed the so-called Uganda Waragi in order to have a conversation. Anyway, I was wrong. I realised that I should not have ventured there. I was to get the right dose of my *'mythical medication'* from her.

During the time I was with my *'mythical niece Enid'* after I had rested, I told her I would need a bit of Uganda Waragi. However, during our chat she asked me how come I had come to Uganda so frequently a few months after the other.

Alas, hell all broke loose! Japadhola says *'Apee!* I met another one that day and curled in my baby-self. She was no-nonsense. She told me that being professional in the medical field she was not going to allow me to take that *'mythical Uganda Waragi'* or any *'mythical alcohol'* for that matter.

And after that, she closed that door of any discussion of having any *'mythical alcoholic thing'* call it whatever name. I cowed into my *'mythical* corner' like a newborn baby and accepted the Jopadhola saying that *'Nyathi goyo buli jadwong bende mielo'* ("A child can also drum and an adult can also dance"). I realised that I had crossed the other side of the Rubicon now being told off and in the strongest terms and unable to strike back. It is the time I accepted to present day now to leave the dance hall to others and to also play their part.

The second time we met again I was told she would be the one to pick me from that *'mythical airport'* and my passport would be confiscated. Hello! *'i'dongo i'ti'*. Hullo!! *'i'dongo i'ti'*. Meaning '...you grow...' '...you get old...'. Such is the new world order, in this *'mythical world'*.

lviii Loss of my *'mythical uncle ASO'*.

When I arrived in Kampala City the following day on the 1st of December 2018, I found my *'mythical uncle'* was in very poor health. I tried to uplift the situation I found, but it was dire. Soon after I arrived within two weeks he passed on. It was a very sad occasion indeed for the family as he was very instrumental in uplifting most people's welfare, name it; especially in education terms. The only thing left to say was for him to rest in peace.

His death devasted my mother who was so close to him for he was instrumental in supporting the sister in our welfare in all ways possible and now he was gone, lying in waste. My mother could not take it as she kept saying "Asaph! What have you now done to me?" I was very scared my *'mythical mother'* would also pass on. But we managed to support her through the mourning process. These are one of the *'mythical scars'* that have scared me.

lix Disclosure to my *'mythical uncle Daddy Sezi'*

During the burial of my *'mythical uncle ASO'*, that is when I disclosed to my uncle my *'mythical Daddy Sezi'*. He had challenges and was weak but he was taken aback as he said he was suspicious something was wrong and was told one time by my *'Mythical sister Nyari Ochido Milyong'* when he tried to discuss with her something and was told not to contact me for anything.

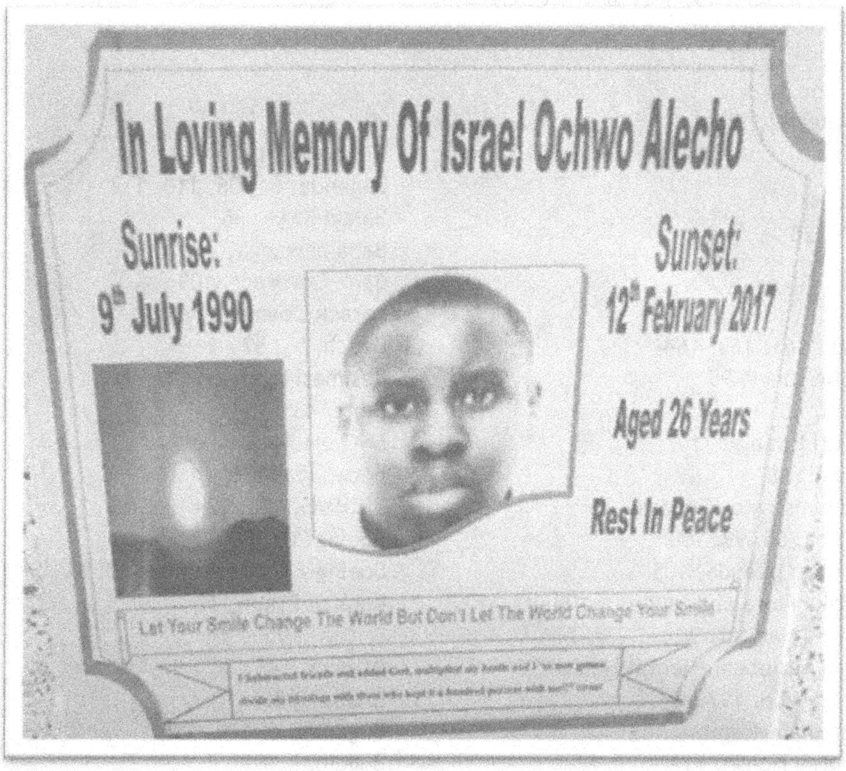
In Loving Memory Of Israel Ochwo Alecho
Sunrise:
9th July 1990
Sunset:
12th February 2017
Aged 26 Years
Rest In Peace
Let Your Smile Change The World But Don't Let The World Change Your Smile

*I wish to draw-in '**My Mythical Tongue**' with a quote from my Late Son Israel Ochwo ALECHO 1990-2017*

"I subtracted friends and added God, multiplied my hustle and I'm gonna divide my blessings with those that kept it 100% with me!!". Israel 1990-2017. RIP

Subject Index

D

E

F

G

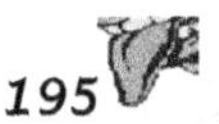

T

U

V

W

Y

Z

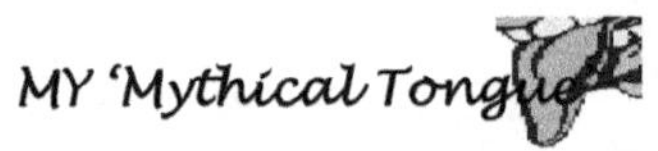

Author profile

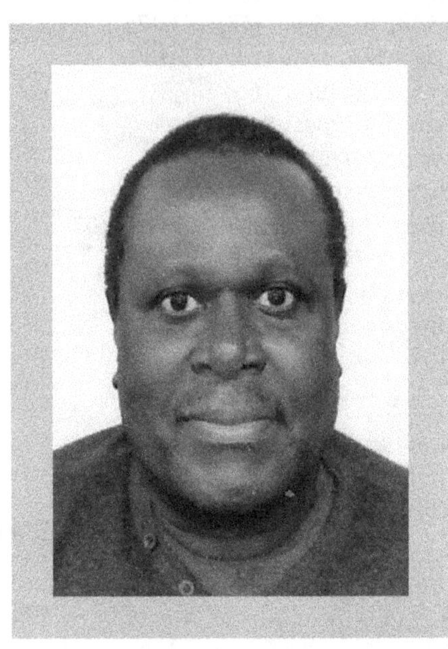

Jesse G S Alecho

Sharper/Brighter / confident Portrait: captured on the 31/01/2018 - after 3 courses of chemotherapy.

Qualifications:

- Postgraduate holder in Housing Management and Practice accredited by The Chartered Institute of Housing [CIH] from the University of Westminster [UK].
- BA [Hons] in Political Science from The Metropolitan University formerly called Guildhall University.
- Diploma in Counselling Psychology from South Thames College; accredited by The Central School of Counselling and Therapy [CSCT].

Gainful living in the UK:

Worked in various fields with the Local Authority, Social Housing and Advice Centre environment. This encompassed; The Royal Borough of Kensington and Chelsea [RBKC], Croydon Churches HA [CCHA], Look Ahead Housing, St Martin of Tours HA [SMOT], English Churches HA, CASYH, Sanctuary Housing, and Citizen Advice Bureau. Afro Caribbean Mental Health Service [ACHMS] Brixton, Oasis Mental Health Project, Merton.

Held various positions in these organisations, such as; Housing Manager, Homeless and Assessment Officer, Housing Officer, Income Officer, Supported Housing Officer, Project Worker, Outreach Worker, Counsellor to name but a few.

Writing:

The writing and publishing of this book have been in part due to what he has expressed in this book; **"My *Mythical Tongue*".** The mystery and/or history of my *'mythical tongue'* arises from his childhood and negotiating his way into social engagement. He was always referred to as *'J'alewe'*, and "*Thombo Nyarienga*" where the mythical tongue sits which reasons for it was unclear to him. He bared and grinned the name-calling. Now, as he faced this challenge of sharing his struggle/fight with 'Cee', the *'J'alewe'* inference writ large in his psychic. So as not to disappoint, he has now notarised *'J'alewe'* ala *'My Mythical Tongue'* as a legacy.

This has brought out the mirroring of reality into myths, like a painter mixing the primary colours of Red, Yellow and Blue to create that '*mythical perfect*' desired shade. This has given him the realisation that had been buried of hidden talent of writing, or to credit his ancestors, they knew it. He has now added a further dimensional interest of exploring writing and publishing further. His mind has gone back into the childhood days when he used to sit out in the night under the clear blue skies in the full glare of the full moon competing with siblings counting the stars and all of sudden there is the shooting star, how sweet that sounds!!

His belief system is that so long as he still feels pain it means he is still alive and capable of exploring beyond the horizon, for pain is the key that unlocks those potentials. Would you follow his '*mythical journey*'? Watch the Space.

To be continued

JesseA

To be continued

JesseA

To be continued

JesseA

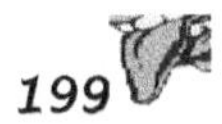

writing [illegible]

[illegible] and publishing of this book [illegible] in part due to [illegible] expressed in the book *My Mutation Tongue?* [illegible] and/or [illegible] my "mythical [illegible]" [illegible] its way into [illegible] engagement [illegible] as a w[illegible] and "Take [illegible]" [illegible] the mythical [illegible] such reasons for it was [illegible] to [illegible] here [illegible] name-calling [illegible] as [illegible] challenge [illegible] this struggle [illegible] *The* [illegible] in the [illegible] as [illegible] discussed [illegible] *My* [illegible] allegory.

[illegible] brought [illegible] of [illegible] scented shad[illegible] of ladde[illegible] further dimen[illegible] exploring [illegible] further. This [illegible] into [illegible] used to sit out [illegible] under the [illegible] in the [illegible] glare of the full moon [illegible] the stars and [illegible] how [illegible]

[illegible] still alive and can [illegible] beyond [illegible] is the key that [illegible] potential [illegible]

To be continued

Jessica

www.ingramcontent.com/pod-product-compliance
Lightning Source LLC
Chambersburg PA
CBHW050118280326
41933CB00010B/1145

* 9 7 8 0 9 9 2 9 4 6 2 9 6 *